Concepts In Kinesiology

2nd edition

D1496730

Richard Groves, Ed.D.
Department of Physical Education
Central Connecticut State College
New Britain, Connecticut

David N. Camaione, Ph.D.
Department of Sport and Leisure Studies
The University of Connecticut
Storrs, Connecticut

 SAUNDERS COLLEGE PUBLISHING

Philadelphia   New York   Chicago
San Francisco   Montreal   Toronto
London   Sydney   Tokyo   Mexico City
Rio de Janeiro   Madrid

Address orders to:
383 Madison Avenue
New York, NY 10017

Address editorial correspondence to:
West Washington Square
Philadelphia, PA 19105

Text Typeface: Garamond
Compositor: Caledonia Composition
Aquisitions Editor: John Butler
Project Editor: Sally Kusch
Copyeditor: Cate Barnett Rzasa
Managing Editor & Art Director: Richard L. Moore
Design Assistant: Virginia A. Bollard
Text Design: Carol Bleistine
Cover Design: Carol Bleistine
New Text Artwork: Vantage Art
Production Manager: Tim Frelick
Assistant Production Manager: Maureen Read

Concepts in Kinesiology 2/e   ISBN 0-03-062372-3

345   090   987654321

CBS COLLEGE PUBLISHING
Saunders College Publishing
Holt, Rinehart and Winston
The Dryden Press

Preface to the second edition

The first edition was designed to assist undergraduate majors in physical education become better teachers and coaches by increasing their understanding of human movement. More recently programs in physical education have broadened their offerings not only to continue preparing physical educators, but specialists in fitness, sport management, sport medicine, and recreation. A review of the literature suggests a strong emphasis toward sport and leisure studies as a major focus in a number of academic programs across the country. Because of this apparent emphasis, the Application section of this text has been extensively revised and concepts developed that deal solely with sport forms. We have attempted to select a variety of sport forms, but more important, to include those that can be easily used to illustrate the many concepts discussed in Sections 1 and 2.

The conceptual approach, which has proved effective in the past, has been retained for this edition. Each concept consists of three parts: (1) INFORMATION relevant to the concept is presented to introduce basic factual material; (2) a RATIONALE which explains the relevance of the concept is presented; and (3) ACTIVITIES are provided for students to complete to reinforce their understanding of the concept.

The selection of concepts for this text was arbitrary. Concepts were chosen on the basis of their fundamental nature and their widespread use in the most popular texts on kinesiology and sport biomechanics. Obviously, total knowledge of this broad subject is not covered. To do so would defeat the purpose of this concise text. We are aware that the selection of the material (and the way in which it is presented) is subjective, but its use for nearly nine years in the classroom has proved successful.

A number of concepts from the first edition have been extensively revised, and several have been deleted. Minor points have been clarified in nearly all concepts. Many of these changes came as a result of suggestions from our colleagues who use the text and from our own classroom experience.

The material is again presented in three main sections—Applied Anatomy, The Production of Motion, and Application to Sport Forms.

SECTION ONE: Applied Anatomy. The format was not altered; only changes and deletions were made.

SECTION TWO: The Production of Motion. This section, which traces the generation of movement in the human body, has been altered substantially. Concepts on Work, Power, and Energy have been added to the beginning of the section. New general concepts before each of Newton's laws were also developed. The Friction concepts have been moved from the Application Section to a more appropriate location after motion, and two new concepts have been added. Three concepts on Projectiles have been included as well. The concepts dealing with Follow-Through have been moved to follow those on Center of Gravity and Stability. The order of these topics now appears more logical and should be more easily understood by students.

SECTION THREE: Application to Sport Forms contains 12 new concepts. We hope this section will provide a practical use of the information presented in Sections 1 and 2. Section 3 attempts to have the student qualitatively analyze certain sport forms using a number of biomechanical principles previously presented. Gaining competence in analyzing a few sports should enable students to transfer these same principles to a wide variety of sport techniques as they gain greater insight and experience in analyzing human movement in sport and physical activity.

This concise text can be used as a single text for a kinesiology course or as a supplement to the sources listed below; materials from these texts serve as the basis for several concepts presented in this book. For your benefit we have listed 16 of the most widely used texts on kinesiology and sport biomechanics.

1.   Barham, J.N.: *Mechanical Kinesiology*. St. Louis: C.V. Mosby, 1978.
2.   Broer, M.R., and Zernicke, R.F.: *Efficiency of Human Movement*. Philadelphia: W.B. Saunders, 1979.
3.   Bunn J.W.: *Scientific Principles of Coaching*. Englewood Cliffs, N.J.: Prentice-Hall, 1972.
4.   Cooper, J.M., and Glassow, R.B.: *Kinesiology,* 5th ed. St. Louis: C.V. Mosby, 1982.
5.   Dyson G.H.: *The Mechanics of Athletics*. New York: Holmes and Meier, 1977.
6.   Hay J.G.: *The Biomechanics of Sport Techniques*. Englewood Cliffs, N.J.: Prentice-Hall, 1978.
7.   Hinson, M.M.: *Kinesiology*. Dubuque Ia.: W.C. Brown, 1981.
8.   Jensen, C.R. and Schultz, G.W.: *Applied Kinesiology*, 2nd ed. New York: McGraw-Hill, 1977.
9.   Kreighbaum, E., and Barthels, K.M.: *Biomechanics, A Qualitative Approach for Studying Human Movement*. Minneapolis: Burgess, 1981.
10.   LeVeau, B.: *Biomechanics of Human Motion*. Philadelphia: W.B. Saunders, 1977.
11.   Luttgens, K., and Wells, K.: *Kinesiology*. Philadelphia: Saunders College Publishing, 1982.
12.   Logan, G.A., and McKinney W.C.: *Anatomic Kinesiology*. Dubuque, Ia.: W.C. Brown, 1977.
13.   Northrip, J.W., Logan, G.A., and McKinney, W.C.: *Introduction to Biomechanic Analysis of Sport*. Dubuque, Ia.: W.C. Brown, 1979.
14.   Rasch, P.J., and Burke, R.K.: *Kinesiology and Applied Anatomy*. Philadelphia: Lea and Febiger, 1978.
15.   Seidel, B.L., and others. *Sports Skills*. Dubuque, Ia.: W.C. Brown, 1975.
16.   Simonian, C.: *Fundamentals of Sports Biomechanics*. Englewood Cliffs, N.J.: Prentice Hall, 1981.

Again, we are indebted to our students and colleagues who offered suggestions to improve the presentation of many concepts in this second edition.

R.G.

D.N.C.

Contents I

SECTION ONE

APPLIED ANATOMY

Planes and Axes   3

Concept 1   Three planes pass through the human body.   5

Concept 2   Human motion is described from the anatomical position.   7

Concept 3   An axis of motion occupies two planes.   9

Muscles   13

Concept 4   The functioning of a motor unit illustrates the relationship between the nervous and muscular systems.   15

Concept 5   Muscles are subject to isometric and isotonic contractions.   17

Concept 6   Isotonic muscle contractions may be concentric, eccentric, or isokinetic.   19

Concept 7   Arrangement of muscle fibers into fusiform or pennate designs determines muscle action.   21

Concept 8   Muscles which span a joint act at that joint. There are single-joint, two-joint, and multi-joint muscles.   23

Concept 9   Muscle fibers are classified into two general physiological types: fast-twitch fibers (pale) and slow-twitch fibers (dark).   25

Concept 10   An inverse relationship exists between the mechanical and physiological advantages of muscle.   27

Concept 11   Muscles may act as "spurt" or "shunt" muscles.   29

Concept 12   A muscle may play one of many roles during joint movement.   31

Concept 13   Human skeletal muscles often play a stabilizing role.   33

Concept 14   Muscles may play the roles of true synergist and helping synergist.   35

Concept 15   Muscles may pull from either direction, a concept referred to as functional reversibility.   37

Concept 16   The brachialis muscle is called the "true flexor of the elbow."   39

Concept 17   Taut hamstrings can limit body flexibility.   41

Concept 18   Three basic hand positions are used to perform chin-ups."   43

Concept 19   For efficient motor acts, muscles must possess sufficient strength, endurance, and flexibility.   45

Joints   **47**

Concept 20   Kinesiologists classify joints according to the degree of movement they possess.   49

Concept 21   Six types of diarthrodial joints exist in the human body.   51

Concept 22   An inverse relationship exists between mobility and stability in human joints.   53

Concept 23   Only three basic movements occur in the human body— bending, stretching, and twisting.   55

Concept 24   Movements at the glenohumeral joint are accompanied by accommodating movements of the scapula and clavicle.   57

Kinesthesis   **59**

Concept 25   Reflexes for skeletal muscles are classified into two main categories—exteroceptive and proprioceptive.   61

Concept 26   The muscle spindle is a proprioceptor.   63

Concept 27   The stretch (postural) reflex is a proprioceptive reflex.   65

Concept 28   Kinesthesis is reinforced by visual information.   67

SECTION TWO

THE PRODUCTION OF MOTION

Work, Power, and Energy   **71**

Concept 29   Work is expressed mechanically as imparting a force over a given distance in the direction of the force.   73

Concept 30   Power is expressed as work per unit of time.   75

Concept 31   Two types of mechanical energy exist: potential and kinetic.   77

Force   **79**

Concept 32   All forces possess specific properties; four are identified.   81

Concept 33   Muscles cause movement at the joints by pulling on bones.   85

Concept 34   To begin a motor activity, a force must be produced within the body to overcome inertia.   87

Concept 35   Desired movement is often the result of the summation of forces.   89

Concept 36   Centrifugal force involves a special application of the law of inertia.   91

Concept 37   Three methods of inducing rotation in an object exist.   93

Concept 38   Force must be applied in the direction of the intended motion to be effective.   95

Levers   97

Concept 39   Three classes of levers are involved in human movement.   99

Concept 40   Certain mechanical factors undergo reductions or gains in lever systems.   101

Concept 41   The elbow joint is an example where all three classes of levers are found.   103

Concept 42   Adding external weight can change the class of a lever.   105

Concept 43   Movement occurs when levers are unbalanced.   107

Concept 44   Identification of the true force arm and the true resistance arm clearly interprets the law of levers.   109

Concept 45   The wheel and axle and fixed pulley machines of the musculoskeletal system are simply special cases of the lever system.   113

Torque   115

Concept 46   Torque is the magnitude of twist around an axis of rotation.   117

Concept 47   Motion can only occur at joints when levers are unbalanced.   119

Concept 48   Muscular contraction (force) results in torque at human joints.   123

Concept 49   A resistance (force of gravity) can cause torque at human joints.   123

Concept 50   Additional muscle force is needed to move a joint when the length of the true resistance arm or the amount of resistance is increased.   125

Concept 51   Forces acting on joints can be divided into two components: rotatory and nonrotatory.   127

Concept 52   Nonrotatory components of muscle force (pull) and resistance yield "undesired" actions.   131

Concept 53   The angle of pull of a muscle changes as joint movement occurs.   133

Concept 54   The angle of pull of a muscle subdivides the total force of a contracting muscle into two components.   137

Concept 55   The human body is mechanically inefficient with respect to force production.   139

Concept 56   The behavior of levers can be explained in terms of moment of force and moment of inertia.   143

Concept 57   Reducing the length of a moment of inertia produces more efficient joint movements.   147

Motion   149

Concept 58   The human body exhibits two types of motion: translatory (linear) and angular.   151

Concept 59   Human locomotion is translatory motion resulting from angular motion at the force-producing joints.   153

Concept 60   A joint exhibits angular motion, while the distal end of a limb may exhibit angular and/or linear motion.   155

Concept 61   A greater linear velocity exists at the distal end of a longer lever.   157

Concept 62   Walking and running demonstrate the alternating action of the upper and lower limbs.   159

Concept 63   Many motor activities involve the principle of continuity of motion.   163

Friction   165

Concept 64   A force that modifies motion is frictional force.   167

Concept 65   In the absence of friction, horizontal movement is impossible.   169

Concept 66   The coefficient of sliding friction is less than that of starting friction.   171

Concept 67   The starting positions for many motor skills demand sufficient friction.   173

Concept 68   Running in sand or mud is difficult.   175

Concept 69   A second force that modifies motion is fluid force.   177

Momentum   179

Concept 70   Momentum is the product of the mass and velocity of an object.   181

Concept 71   Changes in momentum usually occur because of changes in velocity rather than mass.   183

Concept 72   Momentum at the end of a long lever is greater than at the end of a short lever.   185

Concept 73   Motor activities incorporate the principle of transfer of momentum.   187

Concept 74   Impulse is directly related to the concept of momentum.   189

Concept 75   In motor activities in which the body becomes airborne, transfer of momentum must occur at the instant of takeoff.   191

Concept 76   Many motor activities require that a performer reduce the momentum of an oncoming object.   193

Concept 77   Many motor activities require that a performer provide momentum to an object.   195

Newton's Laws of Motion   197

Concept 78   Newton's first law: a body continues in its state of rest or in uniform motion in a straight line except when compelled by impressed force to change that state.   199

Concept 79   Newton's first law: inertia concerns bodies at rest and bodies in motion.   201

Concept 80   Newton's first law: inertia is directly proportional to mass.   203

Concept 81   Newton's first law: a force is necessary to overcome inertia.   205

Concept 82   Newton's second law: the rate of change of momentum is proportional to the impressed force, and the actual change occurs in the direction in which the force acts.   207

Concept 83   Newton's second law: the greater the mass of an object, the greater the force needed for acceleration.   209

Concept 84   Newton's second law: if two forces of different magnitudes are applied to objects of equal mass, the greater force will provide greater acceleration.   211

Concept 85   Newton's second law: the law of acceleration aids our understanding of the law of free-falling bodies.   213

Concept 86   Newton's third law: for every action (force), there is always an equal and opposite reaction (force).   217

Concept 87   Newton's third law: the effect of a performer's action against the earth cannot be observed.   219

Concept 88   Newton's third law: the principle of action-reaction helps to identify the force that propels the human body during locomotion.   221

Concept 89   Newton's third law: the action-reaction principle is observable when a performer is airborne.   223

Projectiles   225

Concept 90   A projectile's path is influenced by certain forces and the angle and height of projection.   227

Concept 91   The trajectory of a projectile involves height, time, and distance.   229

Concept 92   A projectile's path is influenced by impact and the effects of spin.   231

Center of Gravity   233

Concept 93   Understanding the location of the center of gravity in the human body aids our understanding of movement.   235

Concept 94   Each human being has a different specific location for his or her center of gravity.   239

Concept 95   The location of the center of gravity in the body shifts when body parts move.   241

Concept 96   The location of the center of gravity changes when external weights are added to the body.   243

Stability   245

Concept 97   The larger the base of support, the greater the stability.   247

Concept 98   Raising or lowering the center of gravity within the base of support affects stability.   251

Concept 99   Increasing the size of the base of support in the direction of an oncoming force increases stability.   253

Concept 100   Stability and mobility are inversely related.   255

Concept 101   Motor activities exist in which a performer desires to maintain stability.   257

Follow-Through   259

Concept 102   Follow-through prevents a loss of linear velocity at the moment of impact or release.   261

Concept 103   Follow-through prevents injuries caused by the abrupt stopping of a moving body part.   263

Concept 104   Follow-through prevents the violation of certain playing rules.   265

Concept 105   Follow-through provides time to perceive feedback information.   267

SECTION THREE

APPLICATION TO SPORT FORMS

Baseball/Softball   273

Concept 106   Baseball/softball sliding uses the principle of receiving impetus.   273

Basketball   275

Concept 107   The jump shot employs Newton's third law of motion.   275

Downhill Skiing   277

Concept 108   Downhill skiing depends on the force of gravity.   277

Football   279

    Concept 109   One foot must be in contact with the ground when a player kicks a football.   279

Golf   281

    Concept 110   The full golf swing uses an increased lever system to gain maximum linear velocity of the clubhead.   281

Gymnastics   283

    Concept 111   Centrifugal force (inertia) and centripetal force must counterbalance one another during the performance of a giant swing on the horizontal bar.   283

    Concept 112   A floor routine during the free-exercise event uses a number of biomechanical concepts.   285

Ice Skating   287

    Concept 113   A whirling figure skater uses changing moments of inertia to control angular velocity.   287

Starting   289

    Concept 114   There are some motor activities in which the performer wishes to lose stability in certain starting events.   289

Swimming   291

    Concept 115   Effort that does not contribute to the desired result acts as a resistance.   291

    Concept 116   Movement through the water is best achieved by the effective use of a swimmer's arms and legs.   293

    Concept 117   A diver can perform more somersaults in the tuck position, fewer in the pike position, and fewest in the layout position.   295

Tennis   297

    Concept 118   Increasing the length of a moment of force produces stronger joint movements when striking (giving impetus to) a tennis ball.   297

    Concept 119   Follow-through places the body in a "ready position" to begin the next tennis skill.   299

Track and Field   301

    Concept 120   When the body is in free flight, no amount of maneuvering of body parts can alter the path of the center of gravity.   301

    Concept 121   Centrifugal force (inertia) and centripetal force must counterbalance one another during the hammer throw.   303

Concept 122   Hurdlers must minimize their time in the air.   305

Concept 123   The purpose of high jumping is to propel the center of gravity to a height sufficient for good performance.   309

Volleyball   313

Concept 124   The forearm bump pass is an example of receiving impetus (momentum of an object).   313

Concept 125   Spiking the ball is an example of giving impetus to an object.   315

Wrestling   317

Concept 126   The use of levers is important to successful wrestling techniques.   317

Glossary   319

section one
APPLIED
ANATOMY

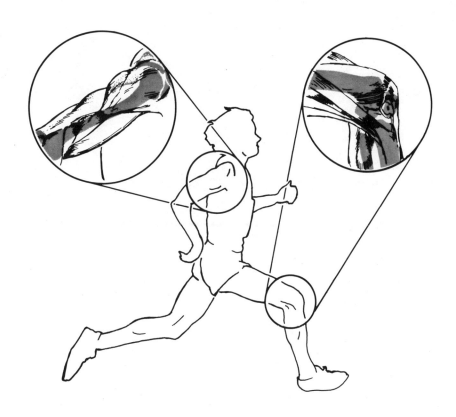

PLANES AND AXES

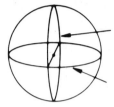 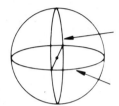 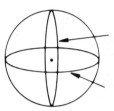

Concept 1:
   Three planes pass through the human body.

Concept 2:
   Human motion is described from the anatomical position.

Concept 3:
   An axis of motion occupies two planes.

PLANES AND AXES

CONCEPT 1: Three Planes Pass Through the Human Body

INFORMATION:

1. In geometry, a **plane** is a level and flat surface which is often imaginary.
2. Three planes of motion pass through the human body:

    a. **Sagittal plane** (anteroposterior): Passes through the body from front to back, dividing the body into left and right portions.

    b. **Frontal plane** (coronal): Passes through the body from left to right, dividing the body into anterior and posterior portions.

    c. **Horizontal plane** (transverse): Passes through the body in a line parallel to the floor, dividing the body into superior and inferior portions.

3. **A cardinal plane** (primary) divides the body into equal portions. The horizontal cardinal plane, for example, divides the body into superior and inferior portions of equal size.
4. The three planes passing through the human body lie at right angles (perpendicular) to each other.
5. Where the three cardinal planes intersect lies the body's **center of gravity**.

RATIONALE:

    Three planes pass through the human body. Human movements are typically described in terms of the plane in which they occur. Axes of motion are described according to the two planes which they occupy. Flexion of the glenohumeral joint may be defined as a forward movement in the sagittal plane around an axis which occupies the frontal and horizontal planes.

    A plane may pass through the body at any point and may divide the body into unequal segments, e.g., the horizontal plane may pass through the body at the ankles.

ACTIVITIES:

1. Complete the following table by supplying the plane of motion in which the action occurs.

ACTION	PLANE
Softball pitch	_____
Sidearm throw	_____
Jumping jack exercise	_____
Flutter kick in swimming	_____
Pirouette	_____

2. In the drawing below, label the three planes that pass through the body.

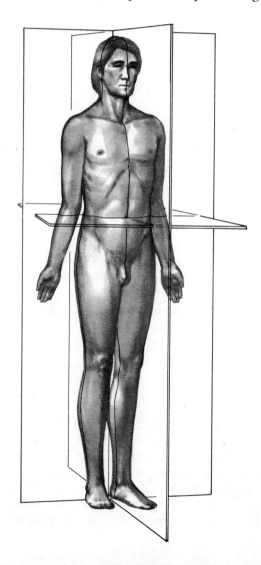

PLANES AND AXES

CONCEPT 2: Human Motion is Described From the Anatomical Position

INFORMATION:

The **anatomical position** is one in which the subject assumes the position of military attention with the palms facing forward.

RATIONALE:

Elbow flexion may occur in different planes. When the arm hangs naturally, elbow flexion occurs in the sagittal plane. When the arms are parallel to the floor with the palms facing upward, flexion occurs in the frontal plane. When the arms are parallel to the floor with the palms facing forward, elbow flexion occurs in the horizontal plane.

It is evident that there must be a standardized reference position from which movements occurring at joints can be described. This fundamental frame of reference is the anatomical position.

ACTIVITIES:

Complete the following table by listing the plane in which the motion occurs. In all cases the person is in the anatomical position.

MOVEMENT	PLANE
Wrist extension	Sagittal
Ulnar deviation	
Hip rotation	

Abduction of leg _____

Plantar flexion _____

Inversion of foot _____

Supination of forearm _____

Anterior pelvic tilt _____

Lateral pelvic tilt _____

Hyperextension of trunk _____

PLANES AND AXES

CONCEPT 3: An Axis of Motion Occupies Two Planes

INFORMATION:

1. An *axis* is a fixed point or an imaginary line about which **angular motion** occurs.
2. A pendulum is an example of an object that exhibits angular motion. One end of the pendulum serves as an axis while the other end describes an arc.
3. Nearly all movements that occur at human body joints are angular motion.

RATIONALE:

An axis is located at the intersection of two planes. The motion occurring around the axis occurs in the third plane. This axis is a straight line about which all mass parts rotate in a plane that is at right angles to the other planes. Three axes are identified in the diagram below. They have been given arbitrary terms, the *x* or medial axis, *y* or transverse axis, and the *z* or longitudinal axis.

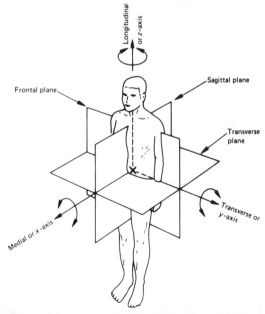

After Dyson, G. H.: The Mechanics of Athletics. *New York: Holmes and Meier, 1977, p. 87.*

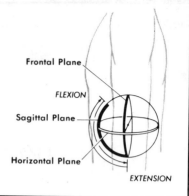

Flexion and extension of the elbow are angular movements. As described from the anatomical position, they occur in the sagittal plane around an axis of motion that occupies the frontal and horizontal planes.

Frontal Plane

FLEXION

Sagittal Plane

Horizontal Plane

EXTENSION

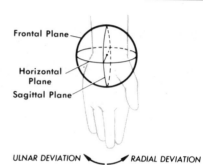

Ulnar deviation and radial deviation occur at the wrist and are movements in the frontal plane. They occur around an axis that occupies the sagittal and horizontal planes.

Frontal Plane

Horizontal Plane

Sagittal Plane

ULNAR DEVIATION   RADIAL DEVIATION

ACTIVITIES:

1. Label the planes occupied by the axes of motion for the following movements.
    a. Flexion and extension of the glenohumeral joint (lateral view).

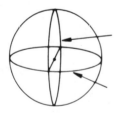

_____

_____

    b. Abduction and adduction of the glenohumeral joint (anterior view).

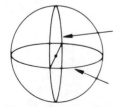

_____

_____

c. Medial and lateral rotation of the glenohumeral joint (superior view).

_____

_____

2. Complete the following table.

MOVEMENT	PLANE IN WHICH MOVEMENT OCCURS	PLANES OCCUPIED BY AXIS OF MOTION	AXIS
Plantar flexion	Sagittal	Horizontal-Frontal	y
Neck flexion			
Supination			
Knee flexion			
Hip extension			
Posterior tilt (pelvis)			
Trunk extension			
Scapula adduction			
Femur rotation			
Trunk rotation			

MUSCLES

Concept 4:
>The functioning of a motor unit illustrates the relationship between the nervous and muscular systems.

Concept 5:
>Muscles are subject to isometric and isotonic contractions.

Concept 6:
>Isotonic muscle contractions may be concentric, eccentric, or isokinetic.

Concept 7:
>Arrangement of muscle fibers into fusiform or pennate designs determines muscle action.

Concept 8:
>Muscles which span a joint act at that joint. There are single-joint, two-joint, and multi-joint muscles.

Concept 9:
>Muscle fibers are classified into two general physiological types: fast-twitch fibers (pale) and slow-twitch fibers (dark).

Concept 10:
>An inverse relationship exists between mechanical and physiological advantages of muscle.

Concept 11:
>Muscles may act as "spurt" or "shunt" muscles.

Concept 12:

A muscle may play one of many roles during joint movement.

Concept 13:

Human skeletal muscles often play a stabilizing role.

Concept 14:

Muscles may play the roles of true synergist and helping synergist.

Concept 15:

Muscles may pull from either direction, a concept referred to as functional reversibility.

Concept 16:

The brachialis muscle is called the "true flexor of the elbow."

Concept 17:

Taut hamstrings can limit body flexibility.

Concept 18:

Three basic hand positions are used to perform "chin-ups."

Concept 19:

For efficient motor acts, muscles must possess sufficient strength, endurance, and flexibility.

Name ————————————————————

Section ————————————————————

MUSCLES

CONCEPT 4: The Functioning of a Motor Unit Illustrates the Relationship Between the Nervous and Muscular Systems

INFORMATION:

1. A *motor unit* is defined as a neuron and the muscle fibers it innervates. Depending upon the type of muscle, a ratio of 1:150 is a normal figure.

2. Where fine coordinated activity occurs such as the hands of a surgeon, the ratio is increased, i.e., 1:10; whereas in gross motor activity, such as a vertical jump, the ratio may decrease to 1:200.

3. Motor units lie close to one another and interdigitation often occurs among muscle fibers.

4. The motor unit functions according to the principle of the "all or none law"; that is, when activated, all muscle fibers in the unit contract maximally or not at all.

RATIONALE:

When one moves a given load (resistance), sufficient motor units have "turned on." If the load is greater, increased motor units come into play, a concept referred to as recruitment.

"Muscle tone" simply implies that a muscle possesses a degree of muscle tension. This tension is developed as a result of motor unit activity. For example, to prevent fatigue, some working units "turn off" while idle units "turn on," thus maintaining a constant state of partial contraction.

ACTIVITIES:

1. Describe the following relationship.

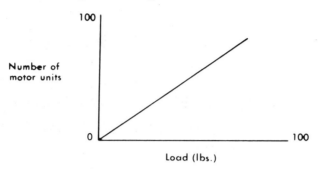

Answer:

MUSCLES

CONCEPT 5: Muscles are Subject to Isometric and Isotonic Contractions

INFORMATION:

Isometric contraction involves no overt change in the length of a muscle; whereas **isotonic contraction** involves overt change in the length of the muscle.

RATIONALE:

Bones move principally because muscles shorten and pull on a bone to which they attach, produce joint movement, and overcome a resistance. This type of contraction is termed isotonic.

In some instances, a muscle may attempt to shorten but cannot because it cannot move a resistance. An example would be a person standing in a doorway attempting to push the sides of the doorway apart. This type of contraction is termed isometric.

During isometric contraction, no resistance is moved because the muscle does not shorten. However, it is evident that the muscle is working (contracting) because heat is produced and the internal temperature of the muscle increases.

ACTIVITIES:

1. How would you counter the physicists' argument that no work is done during isometric contraction because no resistance is moved? ($W = Fd$) (Note: Heat is a by-product of work.)

2. Circle the following statements which depict isometric contractions and underline those which depict isotonic contractions.
    a. Shooting free throws.
    b. Climbing a rope.

c. Pushing outward on a doorway.
d. Propelling a shot put.
e. Executing a pull-up.
f. Shoveling snow.
g. Pulling at the ends of a towel.

MUSCLES

CONCEPT 6: Isotonic Muscle Contractions May Be Concentric, Eccentric, or Isokinetic

INFORMATION:

1. Isotonic contraction involves a change in length of a muscle with the muscle either lengthening or shortening.
2. When a muscle shortens from its resting length, the isotonic contraction is termed **concentric**.
3. When a previously contracted muscle elongates toward its resting length, the isotonic contraction is termed **eccentric**.
4. When the speed of contraction is controlled, the isotonic contraction is termed **isokinetic**.

RATIONALE:

Eccentric contraction involves the gradual lengthening, in a controlled manner, of a previously contracted muscle. A major purpose of eccentric contraction is to gradually lower the body or body part in a controlled manner against the pull of gravity.

A performer arrives at the top of a push-up by means of concentric isotonic contraction of the elbow extensors and scapular abductors. As the body is lowered to the floor, the performer does not allow gravity to exert its full effect, or injury may result if the torso plummets downward. The performer allows the previously contracted elbow extensors and scapula abductors to gradually lengthen (eccentric isotonic contraction) to lower the torso to the floor in a controlled manner.

A major point in isotonic muscle contraction is that the muscle which raise the resistance via concentric contraction also lower the resistance via eccentric contraction.

Modern technology has developed equipment that is capable of controlling the speed of muscle contraction while at the same time producing maximal effort throughout the full range. The Cybex machine used in testing and rehabilitation is an example of such an apparatus designed to monitor speed of contraction. This instrument can be used to control rapid but constant speed against a light resistance or slower but constant speed against greater resistance.

ACTIVITIES:

Identify the following examples as the result of either *concentric, eccentric,* or *isokinetic* muscle contraction.

ACTION	TYPE OF CONTRACTION
Upward movement in a chin-up	Concentric
Downward portion of a chin-up	
Controlled elbow flexion (forearm curl)	
Trunk flexion while standing (posterior trunk muscles)	
Controlled knee extension	
Downward movement in a sit-up	
Elevating barbell above the head	

MUSCLES

CONCEPT 7: Arrangement of Muscle Fibers Into Fusiform or Pennate Designs Determines Muscle Action

INFORMATION:

1. **Fusiform** muscle fibers are those whose **fascicles** consist of parallel fibers running the length of the muscle.

2. **Pennate** muscle fibers are those which have fascicles running obliquely to a central tendon. They give the appearance of a feather.

3. *Fusiform* fibers are generally weak but shorten over long distances, giving the advantage of speed of contraction at the expense of strength.

4. *Pennate* muscle fibers are generally stronger muscles which shorten over shorter distances but with greater force at the expense of speed of contraction.

5. There are several types of pennate structures: **unipennate, bipennate,** and **multipennate.**

RATIONALE:

The human body is designed to produce speed and range of motion. Most of our muscles are designed to produce greater force of contraction to overcome the "inherent weakness" of the body's mechanical design.

The large muscle groups in the lower extremities are predominantly pennate arrangements, and are used for powerful acts such as jumping, sprinting, and climbing.

21

ACTIVITIES:

1. Draw a fusiform, a unipennate, a bipennate, and multipennate muscle arrangement.

        FUSIFORM   **UNIPENNATE**

      BIPENNATE   **MULTIPENNATE**

2. Give the type of fiber arrangement (fusiform, bipennate, etc.) for each of the following muscles. Consider the type of contraction produced by each muscle (see Preface).

MUSCLE	FIBER ARRANGEMENT	ADVANTAGE
Biceps brachii	Fusiform	Speed
Gastrocnemius		
Deltoid		
Quadriceps femoris		
Brachioradialis		
Triceps brachii		

MUSCLES

CONCEPT 8: Muscles Which Span a Joint Act at That Joint. There are Single-Joint, Two-Joint, and Multi-Joint Muscles

INFORMATION:

1. A single-joint muscle acts only at one joint. The brachialis muscle passes only the elbow joint; thus, its sole job is to flex the forearm.

2. A two-joint muscle acts at two joints. The biceps brachii muscle passes the glenohumeral and elbow joints and acts to flex the arm at the shoulder and the forearm at the elbow.

3. A multi-joint muscle acts at several joints. The flexor digitorum profundus muscle passes the elbow, wrist, and several carpal and finger joints. Consequently, it can aid the action of the many joints it passes.

RATIONALE:

A person moves as a result of muscle group action. Research indicates that when several single-joint muscles are used for given joint action, considerably more energy is needed than when fewer two-joint or multi-joint muscles are utilized.

However, multi-joint muscles lack sufficient length to produce effective motion simultaneously at all joints spanned. When the fingers are fully extended, the extensor digitorum communis muscle cannot provide a powerful extension of the wrist. When the wrist is flexed, the flexor digitorum sublimus muscle cannot produce a powerful flexion of the fingers.

ACTIVITIES:

1. For each of the following, find a pair of antagonistic muscles about the same joint(s).

Single-joint muscle pair   _____

Two-joint muscle pair   _____

Multi-joint muscle pair   _____

2. State the actions and the joints involved for each of the following muscles.

ACTIONS AND JOINTS

Triceps brachii   _____

Biceps femoris   _____

Extensor digitorum communis   _____

Gastrocnemius   _____

Brachioradialis   _____

MUSCLES

CONCEPT 9: Muscle Fibers are Classified Into Two General Physiological Types: Fast-Twitch Fibers (Pale) and Slow-Twitch Fibers (Dark)

INFORMATION:

1. **Myoglobin,** a substance having a high affinity for oxygen, is the factor that determines whether a muscle is classified pale or dark.
2. A **fast-twitch** or pale (white) muscle fiber has less myoglobin, less mitochondria, and utilizes the **glycolytic sequence** for energy supply.*
3. A **slow-twitch** or dark (red) muscle fiber has more myoglobin, more mitochondria, and utilizes the **oxidative processes** for energy supply.
4. The human musculature has characteristically mixed fibers within a muscle. In lower animal life, one might find a muscle predominantly fast-twitch (pale) or slow-twitch (dark).

RATIONALE:

Fast-twitch or pale (white) muscle fibers have the capacity to work quickly and derive their energy from **anaerobic metabolism**. Explosive or short-duration activities place great demand on these fiber types. Rapid ballistic actions, such as throwing, shot putting, sprinting, or vertical jumping, use those fibers.

Slow-twitch or dark (red) muscle fibers have the physiological advantage of sustaining contractions over longer periods of time. These muscle fibers are found in posture muscles, those which are under constant stress predominantly from the force of gravity. Activities such as sitting, standing, and walking use dark or slow-twitch muscle fibers. Their contractions are slower and more sustained, but

*Recent research has further subdivided this fiber into two subtypes:
IIA—glycolytic, oxidative, and IIB—high glycolytic, low oxidative.

powerful. Any **aerobic** exercises place great demand on these muscle fibers, e.g., running, swimming, or cycling long distances.

ACTIVITIES:

1. List ten major muscles and indicate whether they can be classified as fast-twitch or slow-twitch (see Preface).

	MUSCLE	FIBER TYPE	TYPE OF CONTRACTION
1.	Soleus	Slow-Twitch	Sustaining contraction
2.			
3.			
4.			
5.			
6.			
7.			
8.			
9.			
10.			

2. From the field of physical education and sports, list five activities that place particular demand upon fast-twitch or pale (white) muscles and five activities for slow-twitch or dark (red) muscles.

FAST-TWITCH MUSCLE ACTIVITIES	SLOW-TWITCH MUSCLE ACTIVITIES
a.	a.
b.	b.
c.	c.
d.	d.
e.	e.

Name _____

Section _____

MUSCLES

CONCEPT 10: An Inverse Relationship Exists Between the Mechanical and Physiological Advantages of Muscle

INFORMATION:

1. **Mechanical advantage** refers to the amount of resistance overcome in ratio to the amount of effort expended.
2. The mechanical advantage of a contracting muscle is greatest when the *angle of pull* of that muscle is 90 degrees.
3. The **angle of pull** of a muscle is the angle formed between the plane of the bone and the line of pull of a contracting muscle.
4. The **physiological advantage** of muscle refers to the ability of a muscle to shorten and can be enhanced by placing the muscle on initial stretch.
5. A muscle possesses its greatest physiological advantage when stretched beyond its **resting length**.

RATIONALE:

If a 10-pound weight is lifted a vertical distance of 1 foot, and 10 foot-pounds of muscular effort are expended, the mechanical advantage is unity (1.00).

A performer hangs from a chin-up bar by the hands with the arms straight prior to performing a chin-up. The angles of pull of the elbow flexors are near zero, resulting in poor mechanical advantages for these muscles. However, because the muscles are stretched beyond resting lengths, they are in a position of physiological advantage. As the performer elevates the body, the physiological advantage of these muscles is decreased, whereas the angles of pull of the elbow flexors increased toward 90 degrees. This demonstrates the inverse ratio of physiological efficiency and mechanical efficiency in the chin-up exercise.

As the angle of pull deviates from 90 degrees, the mechanical advantage decreases. At zero degrees of muscle pull, the mechanical advantage of the muscle is zero; however, the physiological advantage is greatest at this angle.

27

Zero degrees   90 degrees

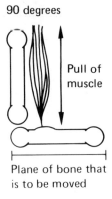

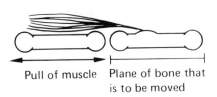

Pull of muscle   Plane of bone that   Plane of bone that
                 is to be moved   is to be moved

Examples of angle of pull, one at near zero degrees and one
at 90 degrees. The first possesses physiological advantage and
the second mechanical advantage.

ACTIVITIES:

Denote by placing a check mark under the appropriate column whether the activity described is more mechanically advantageous or more physiologically advantageous, or an apparent combination of the two factors.

ACTIVITY	MECHANICAL	PHYSIOLOGICAL	BOTH
1. Arms straight, ready to perform a biceps curl with weights.	_____	_____	_____
2. Knees bent at approximately a 45-degree angle preparing for a vertical jump.	_____	_____	_____
3. Legs flexed at the hip at 85-degrees performing an L-seat in a gymnastic activity.	_____	_____	_____
4. Hands hyperextended, ready to perform a wrist curl with weight.	_____	_____	_____

MUSCLES

CONCEPT 11: Muscles May Act as "Spurt" or "Shunt" Muscles

INFORMATION:

1. A **"spurt" muscle** has its upper attachment at a distance from the joint on which it acts and its lower attachment closer to that joint. Example: biceps at the elbow.
2. A **"shunt" muscle** has its upper attachment near the joint on which it acts and its lower attachment at a distance. Example: brachioradialis at the elbow.

RATIONALE:

One factor that determines the amount of force a contracting muscle exerts to move a bone is the distance from the attachment of that muscle to the joint. The greater the distance, the more effective the muscle in moving the bone.

"Spurt" muscles have their lower attachments at a point close to the joint upon which they act and are more effective in producing rapid movement against relatively small resistances. They are effective in rotatory action.

"Shunt" muscles have their lower attachments at a point some distance from the joint upon which they act. Most of their force is directed along the bone and is more effective in stabilizing the bones that articulate to form the joint. "Shunt" muscles also serve as assistant movers when there is considerable resistance to overcome. The role of the brachioradialis in elbow flexion illustrates this assistant mover function.

ACTIVITIES:

Classify each of the following muscles as a "spurt" or a "shunt" muscle. Consult your textbook to identify the attachments of the muscles in question.

MUSCLES	CATEGORY
Triceps (elbow action)	Spurt

Triceps (glenohumeral action) _____

Sternocleidomastoideus (head) _____

Brachioradialis _____

Hamstrings (for hip extension) _____

Hamstrings (for knee flexion) _____

Biceps (for shoulder flexion) _____

Biceps (for elbow flexion) _____

MUSCLES

CONCEPT 12: A Muscle May Play One of Many Roles During Joint Movement

INFORMATION:

1. **Prime mover:** A muscle is a prime mover when it produces most of the force which moves a bone. There may be more than one prime mover involved in a joint movement. Most muscles that span two joints are prime movers of the **distal** joint spanned. Example: hamstrings during knee flexion. ~~Most spurt muscles are prime movers.~~

2. **Assistant mover:** A muscle is an assistant mover when it aids a prime mover in overcoming considerable resistance. Most two-joint muscles are assistant movers of the **proximal** joint spanned. Example: biceps in flexion of glenohumeral joint. Most shunt muscles are assistant movers.

3. **Antagonist:** A muscle is an antagonist when its action opposes the movement occurring at a joint. Example: biceps during elbow extension.

4. **Stabilizer:** A muscle is a stabilizer when it fixes one bony segment so that a movement can occur at a bone articulating at that bony segment. Example: quadratus lumborum muscle stabilizes the left hip as the left leg swings forward when running.

5. **Helping synergist:** Two muscles are helping synergists when they cancel each other's undesired movement, thereby allowing each other's desired movement to occur. Note: when a muscle contracts, it produces all the movements which nature designed it to produce. Some mechanism must exist to cancel out the undesired movements.

6. **True synergist:** A muscle is a true synergist when its movements cancel the undesired movement of a prime mover. Example: the pronator quadratus muscle cancels the tendency of the biceps to supinate the forearm as the biceps flexes the forearm.

RATIONALE:

A muscle may play any one of six roles during a single-joint movement. However, one muscle cannot play more than one role simultaneously during any single movement.

Let us take a look at the actions of the leg muscles. During a vertical jump, the quadriceps act as prime movers in knee extension and the hamstrings at the knee act as antagonists opposing the movement; however, the hamstrings acting at the hip are assistant movers to the gluteus maximus in hip extension. The gluteus medius acts to stabilize the hips during the activity.

In the sit-up, the external oblique muscles of the abdominal group are important in spinal flexion, but each has separate functions to rotate the spine in opposite directions (this second action is counterbalanced), and thus they act as helping synergists.

ACTIVITIES:

Complete the following table by stating the role and action of each of the muscles.

ACTION	MUSCLE	ROLE
Walking	Left quadratus lumborum	Stabilizing left hip
Forearm curl	Biceps	
Crawl stroke (shoulder)	Triceps	
Bilateral leg lift	Rectus abdominis	
Supination of forearm	Triceps	
Batting softball (elbow)	Triceps	
Batting softball (elbow)	Biceps	
Golf drive	Oblique abdominals	

MUSCLES

CONCEPT 13: Human Skeletal Muscles Often Play a Stabilizing Role

INFORMATION:

A muscle serves as a stabilizer when it fixes a bony segment so that motion may occur at a bone which articulates at that fixed segment.

RATIONALE:

In performing bilateral leg lifts, a person lies in the supine position and raises (flexes) both femurs simultaneously. The knees remain extended.

The femurs insert into the acetabula of the pelvis. When the femurs are flexed, the hip flexor muscles attempt to pull the pelvis into a position of anterior tilt. Some muscle or muscle group must contract and fix the pelvis, preventing the pelvis from moving into the undesired position of anterior tilt.

The abdominal muscles, chiefly the rectus abdominis, contract isometrically and stabilize the pelvis from tilting anteriorly. A person unaccustomed to bilateral leg lifts may experience postexercise soreness in the abdominal muscles. The abdominals do not flex the femurs. It is the stabilizing effort of the abdominal muscles which causes the soreness. Unfortunately, this activity often creates problems in the lower back area and is contraindicated as an activity for abdominal muscles.

ACTIVITIES:

Complete the following table by listing the stabilizing muscles. (Consider the movement that gravity would attempt to produce in the stabilized segment.)

ACTION	SEGMENT STABILIZED	MOVEMENT PRODUCED BY GRAVITY	STABILIZING MUSCLE(S)
Chin-up	Pelvis	Anterior tilt	Rectus abdominis

ACTION	SEGMENT STABILIZED	MOVEMENT PRODUCED BY GRAVITY	STABILIZING MUSCLE(S)
Elbow flexion	Scapula	_____	_____
Forearm curl	Wrist	_____	_____
Reverse curl	Wrist	_____	_____
Football punt	Pelvis	_____	_____
Push-up	Vertebral column	_____	_____

MUSCLES

CONCEPT 14: Muscles May Play the Roles of True Synergist and Helping Synergist

INFORMATION:

1. When a muscle contracts, it seeks to produce all the joint movements which nature designed it to produce.

2. *Helping synergists* prohibit one another's undesired movements to permit each other's desired movements to occur. Each synergistic muscle produces the desired movement.

3. A *true synergist* does not participate in producing the desired movement. It merely prohibits the undesired movement of the prime movers.

RATIONALE:

Muscles are nonselective regarding which of their possible movements are produced. When a muscle contracts, it attempts to cause all the movements which it is designed to produce at that joint. Some other muscle acting upon that joint must prohibit the undesired movements.

Two mechanisms exist by which undesired movements may be prohibited. The first is called helping synergy. The biceps femoris flexes the knee and rotates it laterally, while the medial hamstrings flex the knee and rotate it medially. When knee flexion alone is the desired outcome, these synergists prohibit each other's undesired movement (rotation), and each serves as a prime mover in producing the desired movement (flexion).

The second mechanism is true synergy. The rectus femoris seeks to extend the knee and flex the thigh. The hamstrings extend the thigh. When knee extension alone is desired, the hamstrings contract to prevent the undesired movement of the rectus femoris (flexion of the thigh). Note that only one of the synergists serves as a prime mover in true synergy.

35

ACTIVITIES:

1. Helping synergy: The trunk flexors cause the vertebral column to rotate. The trunk extensors also cause the vertebral column to rotate. When swinging a softball bat, trunk rotation is the desired movement. Complete the following table.

DESIRED OUTCOME—TRUNK ROTATION

Muscle Group	Desired Movement	Undesired Movement
Trunk flexors		
Trunk extensors		
Outcome		

2. True synergy: The biceps seeks to supinate and flex the forearm. The triceps extends the forearm at the elbow. When you throw a curve ball, supination is the desired movement. Complete the following table.

DESIRED OUTCOME—FOREARM SUPINATION

Muscle	Desired Movement	Undesired Movement
Biceps		
Triceps		
Outcome		

MUSCLES

CONCEPT 15: Muscles May Pull From Either Direction, A Concept Referred to as Functional Reversibility

INFORMATION:

1. The *origin* (upper attachment) of a muscle is referred to as the fixed point and is toward the axial skeleton.
2. The *insertion* (lower attachment) of a muscle is referred to as the moving point and is away from the axial skeleton.

RATIONALE:

When studying the anatomy of muscles and their attachments it is necessary to learn the origins and insertions. Unfortunately, such learning may lead us to believe that the origins are always fixed points, while the insertions are always moving points.

This reasoning is not always true. In some motor acts, the roles are reversed; the origin becomes the moving point, and the insertion becomes the fixed (stable) point. For example, the sternocleidomastoid muscle arises from the sternum and runs superiorly and laterally to insert on the mastoid process of the temporal bone. Its primary function is rotation of the head. However, if the head becomes fixed, the muscle pulls upon its lower attachment (origin), causing it to move. This action occurs when the individual is breathing heavily and utilizes this muscle as an assistant mover during inhalation.

ACTIVITIES:

If the activity calls for moving the lower attachment toward the upper one, place a check in the first column. If the upper attachment is moving toward the

37

lower, place a check in the second column. (Note: Answer with reference to anatomical position.)

ACTIVITY	L TOWARD U	U TOWARD L
Forearm curl (biceps)		
Sit-up (rectus abdominis)		
Leg raises (iliopsoas)		
Pull-up (biceps)		
Neck flexion (scaleni)		
Forced inspiration (scaleni)		
Dorsiflexion		

MUSCLES

CONCEPT 16: The Brachialis Muscle is Called the "True Flexor of the Elbow"

INFORMATION:

1. The brachialis runs from the lower half of the anterior humerus to the coronoid process of the ulna. It flexes the forearm.
2. The biceps brachii runs from the scapula to the tuberosity of the radius. It flexes and supinates the forearm.
3. The brachioradialis runs from the lower third of the humerus to the distal end of the radius. It flexes, semipronates, and semisupinates the forearm.

RATIONALE:

For the following reasons, the brachialis muscle is termed the *true flexor of the elbow:*

The biceps has a second duty of providing supination, so only when the forearm is supinated can the biceps effectively flex the elbow.

The biceps and the brachioradialis attach upon the radius, thus spanning the elbow diagonally. A poor line of pull exists for elbow flexion.

The brachioradialis has a secondary function of semipronation and semisupination.

The brachioradialis is a shunt muscle, and therefore an assistant mover rather than a prime mover for elbow flexion.

The brachialis is the only flexor that spans the two bones, humerus and ulna, which articulate to form the elbow joint. This muscle has a better line of pull for elbow flexion.

The brachialis has only one function—flexion of the elbow.

ACTIVITIES:

Answer the following questions.

1. Which elbow flexors have secondary functions?

2. Which elbow flexors have poor lines of pull for flexion?

3. What muscle has no other role except elbow flexion?

4. What muscle has the best line of pull for elbow flexion?

5. Which elbow flexor can make the greater contribution to elbow flexion?

Name _____

Section _____

MUSCLES

CONCEPT 17: Taut Hamstrings Can Limit Body Flexibility

INFORMATION:

1. The hamstring muscles have their upper attachment on the ischium at the lower posterior portion of the pelvis and their lower attachment on the tibia and fibula.
2. If the hamstrings are **taut**, the pelvis is prevented from moving into a position of anterior tilt. During the "toe touching" exercise, if the pelvis cannot move into anterior tilt, the pelvis cannot be flexed completely over the heads of the femurs, and the performer may be unable to touch the toes.

RATIONALE:

A popular test of flexibility involves "toe touching." The activity depends upon the ability to fully flex the femurs at the hip. When a poor performance is observed, the investigator erroneously may attribute that poor performance to a lack of flexibility in the vertebral column. In reality, taut hamstrings may be the cause. Slow static stretching exercises for periods of 3-5 seconds repeatedly is the best technique for improving joint/muscle flexibility.

ACTIVITIES:

Execute the following tests for taut hamstrings.

1. Assume a supine position. Raise the right leg from the floor until it is vertical. Repeat, using the left leg.
2. Assume a sitting position on the floor with the knees completely extended. Place the feet against a wall so that the body will not slide forward. Reach forward *simultaneously* with both arms and touch the toes. Do not allow the knees to flex.

3. Go into a deep knee bend and place both hands on the floor, in front of the feet. Keeping the hands on the floor, attempt to elevate the hips until the knees are fully extended.

Each of these three activities is a screening test for taut hamstrings. Inability to perform these screening tests may indicate taut hamstrings.

MUSCLES

CONCEPT 18: Three Basic Hand Positions Are Used To Perform "Chin-Ups"

INFORMATION:

1. The hands are in the **pronated** position when the palms face rearward in the anatomical position.
2. The hands are in the **supinated** position when the palms face forward in the anatomical position.
3. The hands are in the **mid-position** when the palms face one another.
4. Review the attachments and functions of the elbow flexors.

RATIONALE:

In many tests of physical fitness, the performer is asked to execute chin-ups with the hands in the pronated position. There are valid reasons for requiring the pronated position.

When the hands are in the pronated position, the forearm is twisted so that the elbow flexors and supinators are placed on stretch, creating a physiological advantage. The brachioradialis and biceps attempt to supinate as well as flex. For these reasons, the task is enhanced when the hands are pronated. It is the position of choice for climbing a rope ladder without the use of the feet and for scaling a wall. Performing chin-ups with pronated hands increases the ability to perform "real life" tasks.

ACTIVITIES:

Answer the following questions.

1. Which elbow flexor attaches to the ulna, and which does not move as hand position changes?

2. Which muscle makes the greatest contribution to elbow flexion when hands are pronated?

3. Why can the biceps make a greater contribution to elbow flexion when the hands are supinated?

4. Which hand position should be employed when the goal is to develop the biceps?

5. Why is the brachioradialis "exercised" in chin-ups?

MUSCLES

CONCEPT 19: For Efficient Motor Acts, Muscles Must Possess Sufficient Strength, Endurance, and Flexibility

INFORMATION:

1. *Muscle strength* is the capacity of a muscle to exert a pulling force to overcome a resistance one time. One pull-up represents the muscle strength factor for the upper extremities.

2. *Muscle endurance* is the capacity of a muscle to exert a pulling force to overcome a resistance over a given period of time. Two or more pull-ups represent the muscle endurance factor for the upper extremities.

3. *Flexibility* is the capacity of a muscle to stretch or distend about the joints which it passes.

RATIONALE:

Sports educators and coaches have come to understand that the primary prerequisites for efficient human movement are muscular strength, endurance, and flexibility. Other factors, such as neuromuscular speed, reaction time, and balance, appear to develop later when learning motor skills.

Almost all motor acts demand that the individual possess a given degree of muscle development. Some activities place a premium on strength, others on muscular endurance, and many on muscular flexibility. Combatant activities demand a high level of strength; long-lasting physical activities demand sufficient muscular endurance; and flexibility is specific to the activity or muscular group involved. The above understanding is consistent with the concept of specificity of muscle training.

ACTIVITIES:

Rank the factors below for each of the sport skills. (Note: 1 = most important, 2 = average importance, 3 = least important.)

SPORT	STRENGTH	ENDURANCE	FLEXIBILITY
Gymnastics	1	3	2
Football			
Cross-country running			
Wrestling			
Tennis			
Track hurdling			
Soccer			
Distance swimming			
Shot-putting			

JOINTS

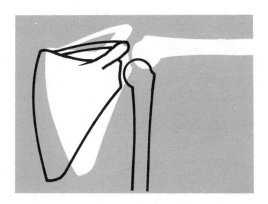

Concept 20:

Kinesiologists classify joints according to the degree of movement they possess.

Concept 21:

Six types of diarthrodial joints exist in the human body.

Concept 22:

An inverse relationship exists between mobility and stability in human joints.

Concept 23:

Only three basic movements occur in the human body—bending, stretching, and twisting.

Concept 24:

Movements at the glenohumeral joint are accompanied by accommodating movements of the scapula and clavicle.

JOINTS

CONCEPT 20: Kinesiologists Classify Joints According to the Degree of Movement They Possess

INFORMATION:

Joints of the human body are classified into three major types—*synarthrodial, amphiarthrodial,* and *diarthrodial.*

1. *Synarthrodial joints* possess no articular cavity and are immovable, owing primarily to their structural unit. Sutures of the skull are an example.

2. *Amphiarthrodial joints* possess no articular cavity but are slightly moveable. The pubic symphysis is an example.

3. *Diarthrodial joints* possess an articular cavity and free movement. They have six subtypes and exist in abundance in the human body.

RATIONALE:

The human body is simply a series of connected blocks, rods, and spheres, linked at points referred to as articulations (joints). Students of human movement must possess a good understanding of joint structure and the resulting freedom of movement.

Certain structural characteristics are specific to the joint type. Knowing these details aids in understanding the particular strengths and weaknesses of a joint. Physical educators are often asked to interpret the degree of movement as they teach sport skills. Structural limitations of a joint or group of joints dictate the style of movement pattern that is to be expected. The significance of joint movement becomes paramount in analyzing total human movement.

ACTIVITIES:

Below is a list of major joints of the body; give the general classification—synarthrodial, amphiarthrodial, or diarthroidial.

JOINT	CLASSIFICATION
Knee	Diarthrodial
Glenohumeral	
Hip	
Vertebral bodies	
Lumbosacral (has a disc)	
Ankle	
Acromioclavicular	
Wrist	
Atlantoaxial	
Coracoclavicular	

JOINTS

CONCEPT 21: Six Types of Diarthrodial Joints Exist in the Human Body

INFORMATION:

1. Enarthrodial joints (ball-and-socket joints) are formed when the spherical head of one bone fits into the saucerlike cavity of another bone; e.g., the glenohumeral joint.
2. Ginglymus joints (hinge joints) are formed when the concave surface of one bone articulates with the spool-shaped surface of another bone; e.g., the knee joint.
3. Trochoid joints (pivot joints) are formed when two bones lie parallel to one another. One bone pivots around its partner which remains stationary; e.g., radioulnar joints.
4. Condyloid joints are formed when the concave end of one bone fits over the convex end of another bone; e.g., metacarpophalangeal joints.
5. Saddle joints occur when two articulating bones have saddle-shaped surfaces which fit into one another; e.g., the carpometacarpal joint at the base of the thumb.
6. Arthrodial joints involve articulating bones that have rough and irregular surfaces. The only movement occurring is a gliding one; e.g., the intertarsal joints.

RATIONALE:

Ginglymus and trochoid joints have one axis of motion and are called uniaxial. They permit motion in one plane. Examples are the elbow, which permits motion in the sagittal plane, and the radioulnar joint, which permits motion in the horizontal plane.

Condyloid and saddle joints are known as biaxial because they permit motion in two planes. They have two axes of motion. Examples are the true wrist joint and the carpometacarpal joint at the base of the thumb. These joints permit movement in the sagittal and frontal planes.

Enarthrodial joints, since they contain three axes of motion, can permit motion in all three planes. An example is the glenohumeral joint.

Arthrodial joints are termed nonaxial because no definitive axis of motion exists. Movement occurs because irregular-shaped bones slide past each other, permitting small ranges of motion in any plane.

ACTIVITIES:

Fill in the following table:

JOINT	TYPE	NUMBER OF AXES
Acromioclavicular	Arthrodial (gliding)	Nonaxial
Hip		
Metacarpophalangeals		
Elbow		
Radioulnar		
Base of thumb		

JOINTS

CONCEPT 22: An Inverse Relationship Exists Between Mobility and Stability in Human Joints

INFORMATION:

1. Some of the factors accounting for stability in human joints are the amount of ligamentous support, the amount of contact between the articulating bones, and the number and strength of the muscles which span the joint.
2. As the factors stated above increase, the stability of that joint increases, but its **mobility** decreases. As the factors stated above decrease, the **stability** of that joint decreases, but its mobility increases.

RATIONALE:

If a joint possesses stability, the amount of ligamentous support, the amount of contact between the articulating bones, and the number and strength of the muscles spanning the joint must all contribute to that stability. However, these factors limit the joint's ability to move, thus decreasing its mobility.

On the other hand, if a joint has limited ligamentous support, less surface contact between its articulating bones, and a small number of muscles spanning it, the joint normally lacks stability. When these factors contribute little to joint stability, joint mobility is increased.

ACTIVITIES:

The hip and shoulder joints are two examples of enarthrodial joints in the human body. These two joints clearly illustrate the inverse relationship between mobility and stability. Answer the following questions:

1. Which joint has stronger ligaments reinforcing it?

2. Which joint has more powerful muscles spanning it?

3. Which joint has a greater degree of contact between the articulating bones?

4. Which joint has greater stability? Why?

    a.

    b.

5. Which joint has greater mobility? Why?

    a.

    b.

JOINTS

CONCEPT 23: Only Three Basic Movements Occur in the Human Body—Bending, Stretching, and Twisting

INFORMATION:

1. *Bending* occurs when the body or body part flexes and confines itself to less space.

2. *Stretching* occurs when the body or body part extends and occupies more space.

3. *Twisting* occurs when the body or body part rotates about its longitudinal axis. (Not to be confused with torque, because all these basic movements involve the concept of torque).

RATIONALE:

Students of human movement are quick to realize that the movements of bending, stretching, and twisting combine to develop into fundamental movement patterns such as running, walking, jumping, throwing, and striking.

Proper motor skill execution depends primarily upon one's musculoskeletal limitations, although secondary factors such as physiological efficiency, attitude, skill, and body awareness have powerful effects in coordinating the movements of bending, stretching, and twisting. Confining one's body parts to limited space or expanding these parts to take up space necessitates coordinated muscular effort if more advanced skills are to be executed.

Thus, the performance of a skillful forward somersault with a half twist to a back handspring demonstrates the combining effects of the three basic movements.

ACTIVITIES:

Classify the following skills as either bending, stretching, or twisting. (Answer in terms of the performer's being in the process of executing the skill.)

SKILL	BASIC MOVEMENT
Tuck forward roll	Bending
Cartwheel	
Pirouette	
Vertical jump	
Racer's start (swimming)	
Bench press	
Swan dive	

JOINTS

CONCEPT 24: Movements at the Glenohumeral Joint are Accompanied by Accommodating Movements of the Scapula and Clavicle

INFORMATION:

1. Each **pectoral girdle** consists of a scapula, clavicle, humerus, and the involved articulations. When one of these bones moves, the other two make accommodating movements.
2. Most of the movements in the pectoral girdle are initiated by the humerus or scapula. The clavicle is not capable of independent movement. If one of the three links cannot move, the range of motion of the other two links is limited.

RATIONALE:

The pectoral girdle can be compared to a three-link chain. When one of the links moves, the other two must make accommodating movements. Otherwise, the primary movement would be inhibited. If the acromioclavicular articulation is injured, the humerus moves with difficulty.

ACTIVITIES:

Fill in the following table. The primary movement is supplied and is marked by an asterisk. The accommodating movements for the other two bones must be provided. For example, when the humerus is abducted, the scapula must rotate upwardly, and the clavicle must elevate.

HUMERUS	SCAPULA	CLAVICLE
Adduction*		
	Upward rotation*	
	Posterior tilt*	
Extension*		
	Abduction*	
Horizontal extension*		
Medial rotation*		
Lateral rotation*		

KINESTHESIS

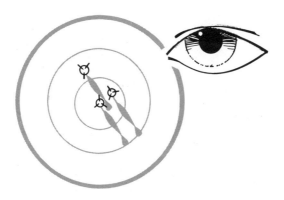

Concept 25:
Reflexes for skeletal muscles are classified into two main categories—exteroceptive and proprioceptive

Concept 26:
The muscle spindle is a proprioceptor.

Concept 27:
The stretch (postural) reflex is a proprioceptive reflex.

Concept 28:
Kinesthesis is reinforced by visual information.

KINESTHESIS

CONCEPT 25: Reflexes for Skeletal Muscles are Classified into Two Main Categories—Exteroceptive and Proprioceptive

INFORMATION:

1. **Exteroceptive reflexes** are initiated by stimuli from the external environment. Examples are the extensor-thrust reflex, flexor reflex, and crossed-extensor reflex.

2. **Proprioceptive reflexes** are initiated by stimuli from the internal environment of our skeletal muscles and joints. The modalities of stretch, tension change, and pressure put these reflexes into action. Examples include the stretch or myotatic reflex.

RATIONALE:

The extensor-thrust reflex is initiated by pressure received in the **cutaneous receptors**, causing a reflex contraction of the powerful extensor muscles in the legs. Merely standing or walking in daily activities elicits the performance of this reflex.

Flexor reflexes are important because they are initiated by pain and protect the body from harm. The hot-stove burn which causes sudden withdrawal of the upper limb is a classic example. This reflex is often referred to as the withdrawal reflex.

A cross-extensor reflex is somewhat more complicated than the other two. However, it plays a significant role in many activities. Protection from pain in one limb withdrawn from the source causes, by way of this reflex, the extensor muscles in the other limb to contract for support. Alternating muscle contractions in the lower limbs during walking, and running use this reflex.

Proprioceptive reflexes are discussed in subsequent concepts.

ACTIVITIES:

Give the specific exteroceptive reflex type (extensor-thrust, flexor, cross-extensor) illustrated by each of the following activities.

ACTION	TYPE OF REFLEX
Blinking when a foreign substance touches the eyeball	Flexor
Jumping as a result of hearing a loud noise	_____
Retracting a foot from the hot pavement	_____
Standing in a line at the bank	_____
Walking into an icy-cold shower (response of the skin)	_____

KINESTHESIS

CONCEPT 26: The Muscle Spindle is a Proprioceptor

INFORMATION:

1. **Kinesthesis** is defined as the perception of muscular movement and the relative position of the performer's body parts in space.

2. The **muscle spindles,** which respond when skeletal muscles are stretched, constitute a major group of proprioceptors that receive information concerning muscular movement.

3. The muscle spindles are located throughout muscle mass and are activated when the muscle they occupy is stretched.

RATIONALE:

One purpose of the muscle spindles is to inform the central nervous system that a skeletal muscle has become elongated (stretched). By reflex action, the elongated muscle contracts.

The muscle spindles control the coordination of muscular behavior. The feedback which they supply assures an appropriate amount of muscular contraction for the task being performed.

One example of the functioning of the muscle spindles is the performance of the "swan dive." The muscle spindles provide the feedback which informs the diver that one arm is stretched to a greater degree than its partner. In the absence of visual feedback, the diver "feels" that the arms are not correctly aligned and is able to correct the misalignment.

ACTIVITIES:

1. Label the following diagram using the information provided.

Muscle   Spindle

Flower spray

Annulospiral sensor

Afferent neuron

Alpha efferent neuron

Gamma efferent neuron

Intrafusal fibers

Extrafusal fibers

KINESTHESIS

CONCEPT 27: The Stretch (Postural) Reflex is a Proprioceptive Reflex

INFORMATION:

1. The **stretch reflex** is generally triggered by the proprioceptors called muscle spindles.
2. The stretch reflex is important in the maintenance of upright posture in humans.

RATIONALE:

Basically, the maintenance of upright posture in humans is a function of reflex action. As the center of gravity of the body drifts toward any margin of the base of support, the muscles in the body segment closest to the center of the base of support become stretched. The muscle spindles in those muscles also are stretched, triggering the stretch reflex.

Action potentials are created in the stretched muscle spindles and travel to the central nervous system (CNS) via an afferent neuron. A component of that action potential returns along an alpha efferent neuron to the stretched muscles. The stretched muscles contract and pull the body mass back into the center of the support base. Stability is regained and the body is prevented from falling off balance.

ACTIVITIES:

You are walking on a balance beam. Your center of gravity shifts to the right and you are in danger of falling off the beam. Fill in the blank spaces in the following paragraph.

As your body shifts to the right, the muscles on the _____ side of your body become _____. The involved muscle spindles also become _____, creating _____ _____, which travels to the CNS via an _____ neuron. A component of this action potential returns to the stretched muscles via an _____ _____ _____. Contractile elements in the stretch muscles contact, pulling the _____ back into the _____ of the base of support. _____ is re-established.

KINESTHESIS

CONCEPT 28: Kinesthesis is Reinforced by Visual Information

INFORMATION:

1. As stated previously, humans possess two general types of receptors specific to skeletal movement; however, one of the most important receptors affecting human movement is the eye.
2. Of the many receptors possessed by humans, the eye is the most significant. In fact, 80 to 90 per cent of our environment is thought to be perceived through visual stimuli.

RATIONALE:

Humans seldom rely upon kinesthetic perception alone. The five major senses aid in reinforcing perception. The diver reinforces kinesthetic information through *visual cues* by looking for the surface of the water while aligning the body for entry; the gymnast pinpoints a visual cue on the ceiling before performing acrobatic skills.

When visual information is reduced or absent, humans as compensatory organisms rely upon the other senses—especially kinesthesis and hearing—in order to maintain balance and posture.

ACTIVITIES:

1. Why are golfers instructed to keep their eyes on the ball during the golf swing?

2. What type of information informs the golfer, prior to contact, that a swing was imperfect?

3. Why do competitive divers request that the surface of the water be ruffled immediately prior to their dives?

4. Why do people recently blinded receive instructions in travel-training (mobility of the blind)?

5. Standing with eyes open, lift one foot to the front and swing the free leg about. Repeat the performance with the eyes closed. Which was easier? Why?

THE
PRODUCTION OF
MOTION

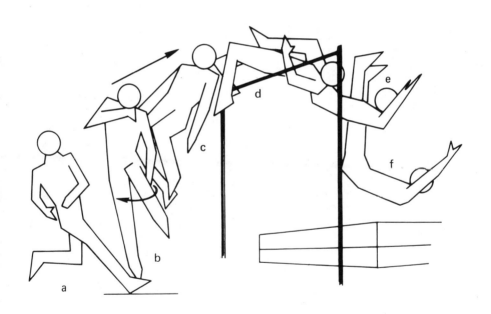

WORK, POWER, AND ENERGY

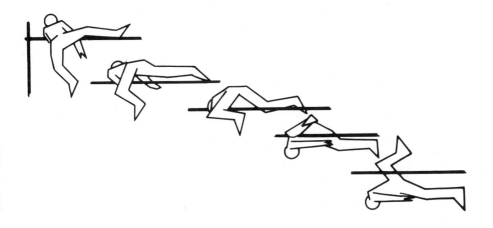

Concept 29:
Work is expressed mechanically as imparting a force over a given distance in the direction of the force.

Concept 30:
Power is expressed as work per unit of time.

Concept 31:
Two types of mechanical energy exist: potential and kinetic.

WORK

CONCEPT 29: Work is Expressed Mechanically as Imparting a Force Over a Given Distance in the Direction of the Force

INFORMATION:

1. **Work** equals force times distance ($W = Fd$). Force is normally applied during a vertical lift (distance).

2. The unit of force used in the English measurement system is the *pound* and the unit for distance is the *foot*; the work unit is expressed as a **foot-pound**.

3. A kilocalorie also is used to express work; it is the amount of heat necessary to raise one kilogram of water from 14°C to 15°C and is equal to 3087.4 foot-pounds.

RATIONALE:

From a mechanical point of view, no work is accomplished unless a force is generated over a given distance. Normally a vertical lift is necessary. That is why it is difficult to measure work that occurs during horizontal movement. Work cannot be computed unless there is a known corresponding resistive force to the horizontal movement. In addition, horizontal movement does not yield a component of motion in the direction of force application.

Examples of work are numerous in sport and physical activity. They include running uphill, jumping vertically to rebound a basketball, spiking a volleyball, high jumping, pole vaulting, leaping into the air during a gymnastic stunt, and propelling objects, as in shot putting, javelin throwing, and ball throwing.

It is often necessary to determine work output when analyzing human performance in order to develop more efficient movement.

ACTIVITIES:

Determine the work output in foot-pounds (ft-lb) and calories for each of the following examples:

	FT-LB	CALORIES
1. An individual lifts a 300-pound weight a distance of 2 feet 10 times for each of 3 sets for a total of 30 repetitions.	_____	_____
2. A track runner weighs 154 pounds and runs a gradual incline, moving a vertical distance of 100 feet.	_____	_____

POWER

CONCEPT 30: Power is Expressed as Work Per Unit of Time

INFORMATION:

1. Work equals force times distance ($W = Fd$).
2. **Power** is expressed mechanically as the rate at which work is performed. ($P = Fd/t$)
3. The unit of power used in the English measurement system is horsepower. One unit of horespower (hp) equals 33,000 foot-pounds per minute or 550 foot-pounds per second.

RATIONALE:

For too long, the word "power" has been used incorrectly to express the work of an athlete in sport events. Muscular explosiveness often is used to describe work performed in a particular activity. In reality, muscular explosiveness is the ability to expend energy rapidly without quantifying the concept. To use the concept of power appropriately, however, the *rate* at which work is performed must be taken into consideration.

The ability to move one's weight over a given distance in a specific time frame in events such as sprinting, executing a number of sit-ups in one minute, and propelling an object rapidly are all examples of power skills. Power is extremely important in many sport skills and physical activities.

If an individual weighing 200 pounds runs the stadium steps, which are a total height of 30 feet, in a 10-second period, the rate of work generated is equal to 600 foot-pounds per second or 1.09 horsepower. An individual weighing 150 pounds performs 10 pull-ups in 8 seconds, moving his or her body a distance of 24 inches during each pull-up; the power generated would be equal to 375 foot-pounds per second or 0.68 horsepower ($150 \times 10 \times 2' \div 8$).

It becomes evident that individuals can improve their power output by either increasing the work output within the same period of time or performing the same work output in a shorter period of time.

ACTIVITIES:

Determine the horsepower generated in the following examples:

1. A person bench presses 150 pounds 30 times in 10 seconds, and during each complete lift the weight moves a distance of 18 inches.
   Answer:

2. An individual weighing 135 pounds vertically jumps a height of 30 inches 8 times in a period of 10 seconds.
   Answer:

3. During a step-test on a 20-inch bench, a person weighing 185 pounds steps up and down 30 times in one minute. What is the power output for the test?
   Answer:

ENERGY

CONCEPT 31: Two Types of Mechanical Energy Exist: Potential and Kinetic

INFORMATION:

1. **Potential energy (PE)** is the ability of an object to perform work by virtue of its position. It is expressed algebraically as $PE = wt \times ht$, where wt = weight and ht = height (distance).

2. **Kinetic energy (KE)** is the ability of an object to perform work because it is in motion. It is expressed algebraically as $KE = 1/2 \ mv^2$, where m = mass, v = velocity. (Note: mass = wt/g)

RATIONALE:

An object has the ability to perform a given amount of work because the object is capable of being raised or lowered against or with the force of gravity. Several examples illustrate the use of potential energy. During a vertical jump, an individual explodes to a height of 24 inches (2 feet) and moves a weight of 150 pounds. The potential energy gained by the person is 300 foot-pounds (150×2 ft). A high jumper elevates the center of gravity to a height of 7 feet and weighs 175 pounds. The PE gained by the individual is 1225 foot-pounds (175×7 ft).

A moving object has the ability to perform work by virtue of its motion. A ball weighing 3 pounds and moving at a velocity of 60 feet per second has a kinetic energy of 168.75 foot-pounds ($.5 \times .0975 \times 3600$). The kinetic energy of a 150-pound athlete running at a speed of 30 feet per second is 2109 foot-pounds ($.5 \times 4.69 \times 900$). It should be noted that KE is directly proportional to the object's mass and to the square of the velocity. Increase the velocity and the KE is greatly enhanced. It is this type of energy which propels an arrow into a target, a javelin into the ground, and a diver into the water with great force (energy).

ACTIVITIES:

1. Determine the potential energy for the following:

	WEIGHT	HEIGHT	ANSWER
Object A	10 lb	300 ft	_____
Object B	115 lb	45 ft	_____
Object C	350 lb	5 ft	_____

2. Determine the kinetic energy for the following:

	MASS/WEIGHT	VELOCITY	ANSWER
Object A	100 kg	50 ft/sec	_____
Object B	200 lb	10 ft/sec	_____
Object C	130 lb	30 ft/sec	_____

FORCE

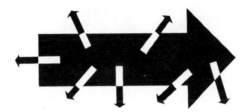

Concept 32:
    All forces possess specific properties; four are identified.

Concept 33:
    Muscles cause movement at the joints by pulling on bones.

Concept 34:
    To begin a motor activity, a force must be produced within the body to overcome inertia.

Concept 35:
    Desired movement is often the result of the summation of forces.

Concept 36:
    Centrifugal force involves a special application of the law of inertia.

Concept 37:
    Three methods of inducing rotation in an object exist.

Concept 38:
    Force must be applied in the direction of the intended motion to be effective.

FORCE

CONCEPT 32: *All Forces Possess Specific Properties; Four are Identified*

INFORMATION:

1. A force has magnitude, that is, the amount of force applied to an object.
2. Forces always have direction; for example, force is applied forward, downward, easterly, or at an angle to the horizontal plane.
3. A force is applied at a particular point.
4. All forces have lines of action or lines of force applied in a straight line.

RATIONALE:

The amount or magnitude of force is essential, especially when the objective is to impart a great deal of distance to an object. Hitting a baseball for a home run or a golf ball 300 yards takes much force. An important concern is always the direction of force. If accuracy is an important consideration, the direction of force must be applied so its line of force is moving through the object toward the intended direction. Therefore, the point of application becomes significant as well. Applying force through the object's center of gravity will result in the object's straight line path, all else being equal. However, if it is necessary to impart spin or curve to the object, then applying force outside the center of gravity will result in rotation (spin or curving).

Magnitude of force

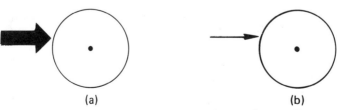

(a)   (b)

Note: The large arrow in (a) denotes greater force; the small arrow in (b) is less force.

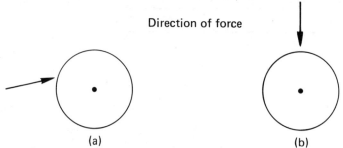

Direction of force

(a)　　　　　　　　(b)

Note: In (a) the force is applied slightly upward; in (b) the force is applied directly downward.

Point of application

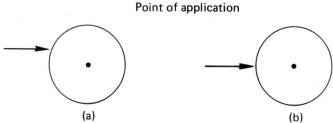

(a)　　　　　　　　(b)

Note: In (a) the point of application is above the center of gravity; in (b) it is going directly through the center of gravity.

Line of action (force)

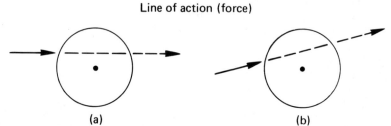

(a)　　　　　　　　(b)

Note: In (a) the line of action (force) is parallel to the horizontal and above the center of gravity; in (b) the lines of force is intended upward and is above the center of gravity.

ACTIVITIES:

For each of the diagrams, place the appropriate line of force.

a.　To lift the object vertically

b.　To tip the object over easily

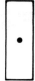

c. To effectively move the object up a hill   d. To push one object further

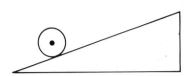

FORCE

CONCEPT 33: Muscles Cause Movement at the Joints by Pulling on Bones

INFORMATION:

1. A **force** is defined as a push or pull.

2. During *concentric contraction* muscles produce force.

3. Muscles pull on bones to cause motion at the joint they span.

4. The **line of pull of** a muscle is along its long dimension or along a straight line between its attachments.

RATIONALE:

Because muscles are members of a lever system, they produce movement at the joints they span by exerting a pull on the bone which moves. The movement of the bone is toward or away from the line of the muscle.

ACTIVITIES:

Indicate the following information by use of arrows in the labeled diagrams on the next page.

   a. Line of pull of muscle.

   b. Direction of movement at the bone.

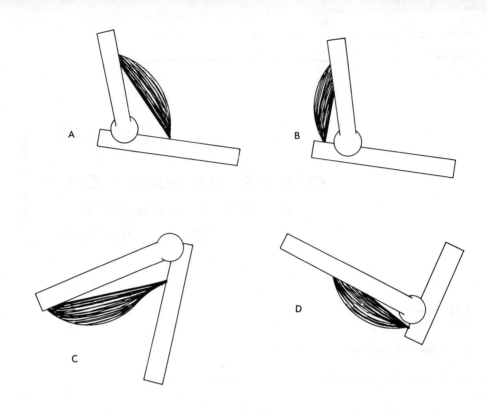

FORCE

CONCEPT 34: To Begin a Motor Activity, a Force Must be Produced Within the Body to Overcome Inertia

INFORMATION:

1. The **inertia** of a body is directly proportional to its **mass.**
2. To overcome inertia, a force must be exerted on a mass.
3. Motor activity involves the movement of the total body or its component parts.
4. The force which commonly overcomes inertia in motor activities is provided by muscular contraction.
5. *Work* = force × distance ($W = Fd$).

RATIONALE:

When a body or a segment of a body is set in motion, the tendency of the body to remain at rest (inertia) must be overcome. To accomplish this end result, a force must be provided. Such force commonly is provided by concentric, and at times, eccentric muscle contraction, which acts upon bones with sufficient force to set them in motion.

Even in events such as diving, in which gravity pulls the body downward, inertia must first be overcome by muscular contraction.

A muscle creates pull by contracting along its long dimension. Typically, muscles contract up to one half their resting length. As a muscle exerts a pull (force) while contracting up to one half its resting length (distance), the muscle accomplishes work and can pull a bone around an axis of motion. The amount of pull produced by a muscle is proportional to its cross-sectional area. A muscle at optimal length can exert a pull of approximately 42 pounds per square inch, or 3 kilograms per square centimeter of muscle.

ACTIVITIES:

A muscle has a resting length of 6 inches. The muscle has a cross-sectional area of 1¼ square inches. The muscle can exert a pull of 42 pounds per square inch of cross section.

How many pounds of pull are exerted by this contracting muscle?

How much work does the muscle perform while contracting?

$$\left(\frac{\text{inch-pounds}}{12} = \text{foot-pounds} \right)$$

What is accomplished by this work?

FORCE

CONCEPT 35: Desired Movement is Often the Result of the Summation of Forces

INFORMATION:

1. The principle of summation of forces can be expressed as "whenever a sequence of movements is employed to impart momentum to an object, each lever must make its contribution at the instant of impact or the instant of release."
2. Levers with the greatest mass possess the greatest inertia and must move first in the sequence.
3. Smaller levers possess less inertia and move last in the sequence.

RATIONALE:

When an angler casts a plug onto the surface of a pond, three levers produce the forces which impart momentum to the plug: the shoulder, the elbow, and the wrist. All three levers must make their contribution at the instant the plug starts forward.

Because the shoulder has the greatest mass, it has the greatest inertia to overcome and must be the first lever to begin to move. The elbow has greater inertia than the wrist and must be the next lever to move. Because the wrist has the least mass, it has the least inertia and is the fastest moving lever. It is the last lever in the sequence to move. In this manner, all three levers can make their contribution at the moment the plug starts forward so that efficient movement occurs.

ACTIVITIES:

1. Five levers that contribute to the momentum of the left fist upon impact with a punching bag are the elbow, shoulder, vertebral column, hip, and the right knee. Arrange these five levers in the order in which they must begin to move.

2. The levers that contribute to the velocity of a golf ball are the elbow, wrist, shoulder, vertebral column, and the hip. Arrange these five levers in the order in which they must begin to move.

FORCE

CONCEPT 36: Centrifugal Force Involves a Special Application of the Law of Inertia

INFORMATION:

1. **Centrifugal force** attempts to pull an object out of its orbit.
2. An object set in motion travels in a straight line (see Newton's first law).

RATIONALE:

The hammer thrower swings the hammer for several revolutions. There is a definite pull on the arms and shoulders as the hammer attempts to escape from its orbit about the shoulders. This pull is centrifugal force.

The physicist argues that centrifugal force is a "false force" and does not exist. The reasoning is that once the hammer or any other orbiting object is released from bondage, it leaves the orbit and travels in a straight line. Such a released object is subject to Newton's law of inertia. Therefore, centrifugal force is merely a special application of the law of inertia. Moreover, centrifugal force is provided by the mass of the orbiting object and inertia and mass are directly proportionate factors.

ACTIVITIES:

1. A softball pitcher uses a windmill wind-up so that the arm travels in one revolution about the glenohumeral joint before the ball is released.
   a. What force causes an outward pull on the arm during the wind up?

   b. Upon its release from the hand, does the ball continue to orbit? If not, describe the path of the ball.

2. A water-skier is pulled behind a boat which makes a wide turn.
   a. The skier feels an increased pull on the arms as the boat begins to turn. What forces causes this pull?

   b. If the skier releases the rope in order to make a landing near shore, will he or she circle around out into the lake or travel in a straight line into the shore?

FORCE

CONCEPT 37: *Three Methods of Inducing Rotation in an Object Exist*

INFORMATION:

1. **Rotation** is angular movement on the part of an object and occurs around an axis of **motion**. The movement is often less than a complete revolution of 360 degrees.
2. Rotation may be induced in an object, including the total human body in one or a combination of the following three methods: (a) by transfer of momentum, (b) vertical **eccentric thrust**, or (c) checking linear velocity (may be termed in some sources as horizontal **eccentric thrust**).
3. It is important to note that rotation in air must be initiated from the ground.

RATIONALE:

During certain diving and tumbling events, the performer wishes to induce rotation in the total body in order to execute somersaults or twisting maneuvers. To accomplish these, the performer moves parts of the body in the direction of the intended rotation. In performing a somersault, the performer flexes the trunk at the instant of take-off. The body, not yet departed from the supporting surface, cannot move in the opposite direction because the mass of the body is still connected to the mass of the earth. Immediately after takeoff, the momentum of the flexed trunk is transferred to the total body which follows in the direction of the flexed trunk. The result is forward rotation, a somersault.

Eccentric thrust involves a force transmitted to an object at some point other than its center of gravity. Batted baseballs rotate because the bat strikes the ball at a point removed from the center of gravity. A thrown ball rotates because the force of the body is transmitted via the hand to a point on the ball other than its center of gravity.

During running, the human body possesses linear velocity. When the toe is stubbed on a rock, linear velocity is checked at an extremity. Rotation is induced, the foot acts as an axis of motion for the total body, and the torso rotates forward and downward toward the ground.

ACTIVITIES:

Complete the following table. An event is listed. Place a check mark in the correct box for the cause of rotation in the listed event.

EVENT	CHECKED LINEAR VELOCITY	TRANSFER OF MOMENTUM	ECCENTRIC THRUST
Diver arches back at takeoff		✓	
Batted ball exhibits topspin			
Runner trips on hurdle			
"Hooked" golf ball			
High jumper leans back as takeoff foot is planted			
Hopping fastball pitch in baseball			
Turntable on trampoline			
Double forward somersault dive			
Boy stubs toe—lands on face			
Backspin on golf shot			

FORCE

CONCEPT 38: Force Must be Applied in the Direction of the Intended Motion to be Effective

INFORMATION:

1. A force can be subdivided into components.

2. Force applied through the center of gravity causes an object to travel in a straight line.

RATIONALE:

A right-handed golfer swings diagonally at a ball, which travels down the fairway a short distance, landing in the right rough.

The explanation is not all of the force provided by the moving clubhead was applied in the intended direction, straight down the fairway. The diagonal swing caused the force of the clubhead to be divided into two components, forward and lateral. Because the ball moved laterally to the right, it could not travel as far forward as would be the case if all the force had been applied in the intended direction.

ACTIVITIES:

1. A person is pushing a heavy box across the floor. Muscular force is exerted in the direction indicated by the arrow in the diagram on page 96.

a. Draw dotted-line arrows indicating the two components of force.
b. Which component represents unnecessary work and, in turn, increases the difficulty of the task?

c. Indicate by a solid-line arrow the direction in which the person should have applied the force.

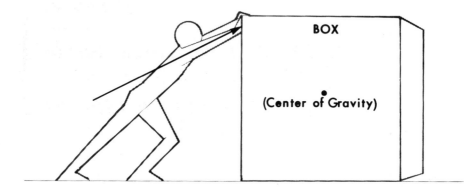

2. A baseball pitcher who throws a curve ball supinates the forearm during the pitching motion to impart spin to the ball. In light of the information presented in this concept, why is it difficult for a pitcher to throw a curve ball with a velocity equal to that of a fast ball?

LEVERS

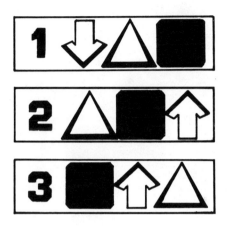

Concept 39:
Three classes of levers are involved in human movement.

Concept 40:
Certain mechanical factors undergo reductions or gains in lever systems.

Concept 41:
The elbow joint is an example where all three classes of levers are found.

Concept 42:
Adding external weight can change the class of a lever.

Concept 43:
Movement occurs when levers are unbalanced.

Concept 44:
Identification of the true force arm and the true resistance arm clearly interprets the law of levers.

Concept 45:
The wheel and axle and fixed pulley machines of the musculoskeletal system are simply special cases of the lever system.

LEVERS

CONCEPT 39: Three Classes of Levers are Involved in Human Movement

INFORMATION:

1. A **lever** is a simple machine. A resistance is moved through a distance. A lever produces work.
2. The three parts of a lever are the **force point** (the exact point where the effort is applied), the **resistance point** (the exact point on which the resistance acts), and the **fulcrum** (the axis of motion).
3. The *resistance point* in a human body lever frequently is the center of gravity of the moving body segment plus any external weights.
4. The **force arm** of a lever is the distance from the force point to the *axis of motion* (fulcrum).
5. The **resistance arm** of a lever is the distance from the resistance point to the *axis of motion.*
6. The relative arrangement of the force point, resistance point, and fulcrum distinguishes the three classes of levers.

RATIONALE:

A lever is a machine capable of performing work. Effort (force) is applied at one point, and a resistance at some other point is moved. The lever pivots about an axis of motion called the fulcrum.

A **first-class lever** has its fulcrum at some location between the resistance point and the force point. Example: see-saw. A **second-class lever** has its resistance point at some location between the force point and the fulcrum. Example: wheelbarrow. **A third-class lever** has its force point at some location between the resistance point and the fulcrum. Example: shovel.

A body part that moves acts as a lever. The joint (fulcrum) is the fixed axis of motion about which *angular motion* occurs. The force is provided by a contracting muscle and the insertion of that muscle into the moving bone is the force point. The resistance in the system is commonly the pull of gravity. The resistance point is the center of gravity of the moving body segment plus any external objects attached to that segment.

ACTIVITIES:

1. Draw and label the three classes of levers.
    a.

    b.

    c.

LEVERS

CONCEPT 40: Certain Mechanical Factors Undergo Reductions or Gains in Lever Systems

INFORMATION:

1. Different lever classes provide increases or decreases in three mechanical factors: force, speed of movement, and range of motion.
2. A reduction in one of these factors is accompanied by a gain in one or both of the remaining factors.
3. The relative lengths of the force arm and the resistance arm aid in understanding which factors are improved or reduced.
4. All of the above statements are in accord with one of the most fundamental physical laws, the conservation of energy, which states that energy can be neither created nor destroyed but may change its form; that is, energy is conserved.

RATIONALE:

When a simple machine such as a lever is employed, certain factors are either gained or reduced. If a first-class lever has a force arm longer than its resistance arm, a gain in force will result. However, there will be an accompanying reduction in range and speed of motion. The resistance arm moves a shorter distance than the force arm and moves closer.

A second-class lever always has a longer force arm than its resistance arm. This class of lever produces a gain in force. More resistance can be overcome than force applied but the resistance arm moves slower through a shorter range of motion. Because a greater force arm exists, less force is needed to overcome a greater resistance.

The third-class lever always has a resistance arm longer than its force arm. Such levers suffer a reduction in force. A relatively light resistance is moved rapidly through a longer range of motion because the amount of force applied exceeds the amount of resistance moved.

When a first-class lever has a longer resistance arm than its force arm, there will be a reduction in force. However, a gain in range and speed of motion will be realized. Should a force greater than the resistance be applied to such a lever, the resistance arm will move rapidly through a range of motion greater than that of the force arm.

ACTIVITIES:

Study each diagram and identify the class of lever. Write in the factor(s) gained or reduced in each diagram.

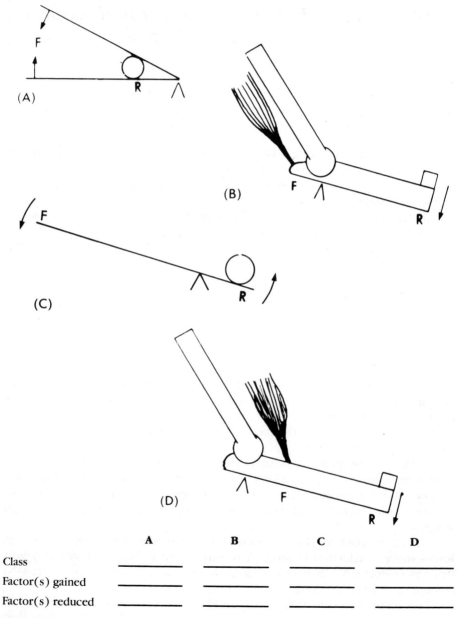

	A	B	C	D
Class	_____	_____	_____	_____
Factor(s) gained	_____	_____	_____	_____
Factor(s) reduced	_____	_____	_____	_____

LEVERS

CONCEPT 41: The Elbow Joint is an Example Where all Three Classes of Levers are Found

INFORMATION:

1. A human body lever may consist of one or more moving bones (resistance), a joint (axis of motion), and one or more contracting muscles (force).

2. The *resistance point* of a body segment is normally 3/7 of the distance from the proximal end when no external weights are attached.

3. It is possible to demonstrate that different levers can exist at the same joint.

RATIONALE:

Three primary flexor muscles and one primary extensor muscle move the forearm at the elbow. The elbow is the axis and the forearm is the resistance.

Elbow extension involves a first-class lever. The triceps inserts (force point) onto the olecranon process of the ulna which protrudes above the joint. The center of gravity (resistance point) of the forearm is 3/7 of the distance from the joint to the finger tips. Thus, a force, fulcrum, and resistance relationship exists.

The action of the brachioradialis muscle at the elbow joint serves as a second-class lever. The muscle inserts (force point) into the radius at a point beyond the resistance point (center of gravity). Thus, a fulcrum, resistance, and force relationship exists.

Both the biceps and the brachialis muscles act to construct a third-class lever. They insert into the forearm at points that are between the joint (axis) and the center of gravity (resistance point). Thus, a fulcrum, force, and resistance relationship exists.

ACTIVITIES:

Label the following diagram. Draw in the approximate muscle attachments and indicate the location of the force point, resistance point, and fulcrum. Classify the type of lever involved and indicate the factors gained or reduced.

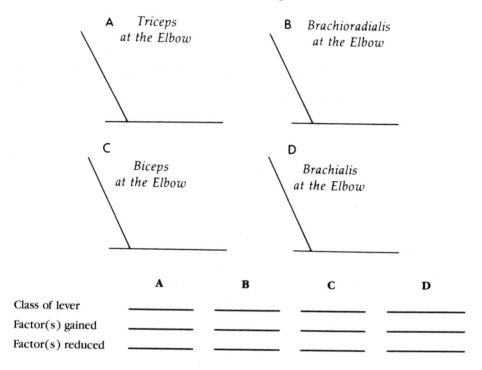

	A	**B**	**C**	**D**
Class of lever				
Factor(s) gained				
Factor(s) reduced				

LEVERS

CONCEPT 42: Adding External Weight Can Change the Class of a Lever

INFORMATION:

1. Levers are classified according to the relative location of the force point, resistance point, and fulcrum.
2. Adding external weights to a body segment can cause a shift in the location of its center of gravity (resistance point), which could result in a change in the class of lever.

RATIONALE:

The brachioradialis muscle inserts into (force point) the styloid process, located near the distal end of the radius. The center of gravity of the forearm (resistance point) is between the force point and the joint when the hands are empty. The brachioradialis serves as a second-class lever.

When external weight is held in the hands, the center of gravity of the forearm shifts toward the hands. If the weight is sufficient, the center of gravity shifts to a point beyond the insertion of the brachioradialis. The class of lever for the brachioradialis muscle now shifts from second- to third-class. It is the change in the position of the resistance point that is responsible for this shift.

ACTIVITIES:

Consider the following drawings. Locate the position of the fulcrum, the force point, and the resistance point in each drawing. Classify the type of lever involved and indicate the factors gained or reduced.

A

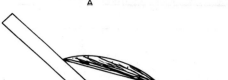

Hands empty

B

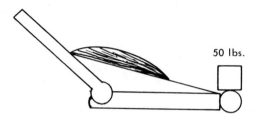

50 lbs.

External weight in hands

	A	**B**
Class of lever	————————	————————
Factor(s) gained	————————	————————
Factor(s) reduced	————————	————————

LEVERS

CONCEPT 44: Identification of the True Force Arm and the True Resistance Arm Clearly Interprets the Law of Levers

INFORMATION:

1. **Torque** is a lever action that uses the joint as an axis, with muscles providing the force and body segments or external weights providing the resistance.
2. The **true force arm** is defined as the **perpendicular** distance from the **line of pull of the muscle** to the axis of motion (the joint). The line of pull of a muscle lies in a straight line between its two attachments.
3. The **true resistance arm** is defined as the *perpendicular* distance from the *line of pull of the resistance* to the axis of motion (the joint). The line of pull of resistance ordinarily is a vertical line.
4. The amount of torque occurring at a joint can be measured when the following factors are known:

   a. the amount of force applied to the bone
   b. the length of the true force arm
   c. the amount of resistance to be overcome
   d. the length of the true resistance arm

5. The law of levers should be amended to read that a lever is balanced when force times true force arm equals resistance times true resistance arm. ($F \times TFA = R \times TRA$.)

RATIONALE:

The law of levers stated in the prior concept is oversimplified. Consider two children operating a seesaw with the plank that Child A sits on being too short to rest on the ground.

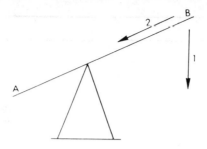

In this case, all of the force produced by the weight of Child B does not move the child downward. Only a portion of the force moves Child B downward (1), while another force is directed along the plank (2) and would, if great enough, shear the bolt holding the plank to the fulcrum. Consequently, this demonstrates that only a portion of the force in a lever system produces the desired motion (Child B moving downward).

In the previous concept, the force arm and the resistance arm were measured along the lever (see below).

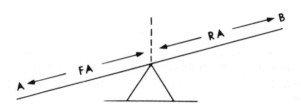

All of the force produced by gravity acting on Child B is not used to produce the desired motion. Some was lost because it was directed along the plank toward the fulcrum.

The amended law of levers includes the true force arm and the true resistance arm necessary for producing torque. The diagram below represents an interpretation of the *true force arm* (CD).

B represents the force point, C the axis of rotation, and the dotted line (CD) represents the true force arm. It is apparent, when measured, that line CD is shorter than BC or that the true force arm is shorter than the force arm. The true force arm thus represents the component of force that provides motion at the fulcrum (joint). Child A represents the resistance, line AC the resistance arm, and line CE the *true resistance arm*. As in the force arms, the true resistance arm is shorter than the resistance arm. Thus, not all the force (weight of Child A) is directed to the desired outcome, causing Child A's end of the plank to descend further.

110

ACTIVITIES:

1. Draw the true force arm and the true resistance arm in the following muscle diagram.

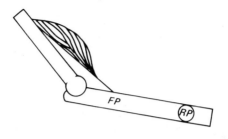

2. Torque provided by a contracting muscle is determined by multiplying $F \times TFA$, resulting in units of foot-pounds. In the drawing for activity 1, the force = 200 pounds and the $TFA = 1/2$ inch. What amount of torque is produced in the system to flex the forearm at the elbow (in foot-pound units)?
Answer:

3. A heavy resistance also can cause a lever to move downward. Example: a heavy weight can cause a flexed elbow to extend. Torque provided by a resistance is determined by multiplying $R \times TRA$. In activity 2, if R = 50 pounds and $TRA = 15$ inches, what is the amount of torque producing extension at the elbow?
Answer:

LEVERS

CONCEPT 45: The Wheel and Axle and Fixed Pulley Machines of the Musculoskeletal System are Simply Special Cases of the Lever System

INFORMATION:

1. When force is applied to an axle, the force arm is shortened and force is sacrificed for speed; however, when force is applied to the wheel, the force arm is lengthened and speed is sacrificed for force.
2. The sliding of a tendon around a prominent marking establishes a first-class lever system. This machine acts to change the direction of the line of pull of a muscle in addition to increasing its angle of pull.

RATIONALE:

Like most other levers in the body, the wheel and axle is utilized to gain speed and range of motion at the expense of force. The twisting or rotatory movements about the longitudinal axis of a bony part are examples of this simple machine action. Investigation demonstrates that we possess both types where force is applied to the rim and where force is applied to the axle.

The fixed pulley is often found in the musculoskeletal system. Two important events occur in the fixed pulley. As the line of pull of a muscle is changed, the angle of pull increases, and the true force arm increases. Diagram A illustrates an increased true force arm; Diagram B illustrates an increased angle of pull.

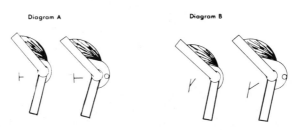

Diagram A   Diagram B

ACTIVITIES:

1. Describe two wheel and axle machines within the human body, one with force applied to the wheel and the other with the force applied to the axle.

   a.

   b.

2. Cite five muscles whose tendons turn about a prominent bony marking and develop into a fixed pulley system.

   a.

   b.

   c.

   d.

   e.

TORQUE

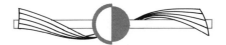

Concept 46:
Torque is the magnitude of twist around an axis of motion.

Concept 47:
Motion can only occur at joints when levers are unbalanced.

Concept 48:
Muscular contraction (force) results in torque at human joints.

Concept 49:
A resistance (force of gravity) can cause torque at human joints.

Concept 50:
Additional muscle force is needed to move a joint when the length of the true resistance arm or the amount of resistance is increased.

Concept 51:
Forces acting on joints can be divided into two components: rotatory and nonrotatory.

Concept 52:
Nonrotatory components of muscle force (pull) and resistance yield "undesired" actions.

Concept 53:
The angle of muscle pull changes as joint movement occurs.

Concept 54:
The angle of pull of a muscle subdivides the total force of a contracting muscle into two components.

Concept 55:
The human body is mechanically inefficient with respect to force production.

Concept 56:

The behavior of levers can be explained in terms of moment of force and moment of inertia.

Concept 57:

Reducing the length of a moment of inertia produces more efficient joint movements.

TORQUE

CONCEPT 46: Torque is the Magnitude of Twist Around an Axis of Rotation

INFORMATION:

1. *Torque* or twist can be rotatory (angular) movement in any plane about an axis of motion.

2. To more clearly understand torque, *force* will be continuously used interchangeably with muscular contraction, while *resistance* will be the pull of gravity, the opposing force.

3. Torque occurs when bones move around each other at joints which serve as axes of movement.

RATIONALE:

Torque occurs when bones move at joints. For example, when flexing the elbow, the proximal end of the ulna rotates around the spool-shaped distal end of the humerus. When abducting the arm at the shoulder, the humerus follows a rotatory (angular) path within the glenoid fossa of the scapula. Thus, the angular motion of a bone moving around a joint falls within the definition and understanding of torque.

ACTIVITIES:

Column 1 has a list of activities occurring in daily life. Place a "Yes" in column II if the activity is an example of torque. If the answer for column II is "Yes," enter the axis of motion in column III.

I Activity	II Torque Yes or No	III Axis of Motion
Working a woodscrew into a plank	Yes	Long axis of woodscrew
Pulling a nail from a plank		
Wringing out a wet towel		
Extending the elbow		
Stepping on an automobile gas pedal		
Riding down a rollercoaster		
Turning on the TV		
Standing at attention		
Shoulder action in forehand tennis stroke		
Chewing gum		
Drinking through a straw		

TORQUE

CONCEPT 47: Motion Can Only Occur at Joints When Levers are Unbalanced

INFORMATION:

1. *Torque* is the product of a force transmitted across a perpendicular distance from the line of action.

2. Either the pull of a contracting muscle or the pull of some resistance can result in torque.

RATIONALE:

Motion can occur at a joint only when the involved lever is unbalanced. When the lever is balanced, no motion results at the joint.

Using the elbow joint as an example, let us consider the arm in the anatomical position. The elbow can be flexed only when the torque produced by the contracting elbow flexors ($F \times TFA$) is greater than the torque produced by the weight of the forearm ($R \times TRA$).

In the same manner, the pull of gravity can move the flexed elbow into extension only when the torque produced by $R \times TRA$ exceeds the torque produced by the elbow flexors; that is, if we can "partial out" the phenomenon of eccentric contraction of the elbow flexors.

ACTIVITIES:

1. Diagnose the following torque situation. A subject in the **supine** position is attempting to hold a bilateral leg lift position.

    > GIVEN:
    > $F = 500$ lb
    > $TFA = 2$ in
    > $R = 50$ lb
    > $TRA = 15$ in

    Will the legs continue to rise through flexion, or will they drop to the floor?

2. Complete the following table. Columns I and II list the possible movements. Columns III, IV, V, and VI provide necessary data. In column VII, list the movement from column I or II, which, in fact, does occur.

I	II	III	IV	V	VI	VII
Motion Caused by Force	Motion Caused by Resistance	F	TFA	R	TRA	Resulting Motion
Elbow flexion	Elbow extension	50	1″	15	9″	Extension
Wrist flexion	Wrist extension	25	1½″	3	3″	
Arm abduction	Arm adduction	100	2″	15	15″	
Dorsiflexion	Plantar flexion	200	3″	5	6″	

TORQUE

CONCEPT 48: Muscular Contraction (Force) Results in Torque at Human Joints

INFORMATION:

1. The amount of torque produced by a contracting muscle is determined by multiplying the amount of force (pounds) developed by the contracting muscle(s) by the length of the *true force arm*. The answer is expressed in units of foot-pounds.

2. When a muscle contracts to cause motion at a joint, the pull produced by the muscle is transmitted across perpendicular distance to the involved joint, and the resulting torque produces angular motion.

RATIONALE:

Movements occurring at joints are the result of torque. The force causing movements at joints is commonly the result of *concentric contraction.*

The longer the true force arm, the greater the amount of torque available to produce motion. This becomes obvious when a mechanic selects a long-handled wrench to remove a rusty bolt. Unfortunately, muscles in the human body attach themselves to bones in close proximity to the joints, resulting in short true force arms. As a consequence, a lesser amount of torque is produced for the desired angular motion. Therefore, much of the pull of the muscle may be expended in serving some other purpose.

ACTIVITIES:

1. Complete the following table. Column I lists a constant force of 300 pounds of pull produced by a contracting muscle. Column II lists varying true force arms. (Note: Convert inches to decimal portions of one foot.) In Column III, list the amount of torque in foot-pounds that is produced to move the joint.

I	II	III
Force	TFA	Torque Produced
300 lb	⅛" (.01 feet)	3 ft-lb
300 lb	¼"	
300 lb	½"	
300 lb	¾"	
300 lb	1"	
300 lb	1½"	

2. For activity 1, answer the following.

    a. Which *TFA* produced the least torque?

    b. Which *TFA* produced the most torque?

    c. Explain the relationship that exists between the length of *TFA* and the amount of torque produced.

TORQUE

CONCEPT 49: A Resistance (Force of Gravity) Can Cause Torque at Human Joints

INFORMATION:

1. A heavy resistance can produce enough torque to cause the joints to move. When the abducted arm is subjected to the pull of gravity, the extremity will become adducted.

2. When gravity or some other resistance pulls on a body segment, the resistive force is transmitted across a perpendicular distance (*true resistance arm*) to the involved joint and the resulting torque produces motion.

RATIONALE:

Many human movements occur, in part or in whole, when some resistance causes a body segment to move at a joint. A commonly employed resistive force is gravity. Gravity exerts all of its force in a vertical direction on the center of gravity (resistance point) of the body segment. If no external weights are added to a body segment, its resistance point is located 3/7 of the distance from the proximal end.

The resistive force is transmitted across a perpendicular distance (true resistance arm) to the involved joint. Torque is produced, and motion occurs. The longer the true resistance arm, the greater the quantity of torque produced. A weight at the end of a longer lever will swing down faster than the same weight at the end of a shorter lever.

Unfortunately, in the human body the true resistance arms typically are longer than the true force arms. The torque produced by the resistance is considerable. Therefore, the muscle must produce great amounts of pull to lift relatively light resistances.

ACTIVITIES:

1. Complete the following table. Column I lists a constant resistance of 100 pounds. Column II lists varying true resistance arms. In column III, list the amount of torque that is produced at the joint in foot-pounds.

I	II	III
Resistance	TRA	Torque Produced
100 lb	7" (.58 ft)	58 ft-lb
100 lb	8"	
100 lb	9"	
100 lb	10"	
100 lb	11"	
100 lb	12"	

2. Questions regarding activity 1.

   a. Which *TRA* produced the least torque?

   b. Which *TRA* produced the most torque?

   c. What type of relationship exists between the length of the *TRA* and the amount of torque produced?

TORQUE

CONCEPT 50: Additional Muscle Force is Needed to Move a Joint When the Length of the True Resistance Arm or the Amount of Resistance is Increased

INFORMATION:

1. The *torque* produced by a resistance is the product of the amount of resistance multiplied by the length of the true *resistance arm*.
2. If an external weight is added to a body segment, the center of gravity (*resistance point*) shifts toward the location of that external weight.
3. A weight added to the hand, therefore, increases the resistance (weight) of the arm and lengthens the true resistance arm.

RATIONALE:

It is easier to raise a balky window by standing close, rather than at arm's length, because the length of the resistance arm is short when standing near the window.

Whenever a heavy weight must be lifted, the center of gravity of the person doing the lifting is moved as close as possible to the weight. As a consequence, the true resistance arm is made shorter so that the muscle effort (force) is directed primarily to the desired goal of lifting the weight as efficiently as possible.

ACTIVITIES:

1. **Situation A.** The deltoid is flexing the humerus and the hands are empty. The glenohumeral joint is the axis of motion. Using the formula $F \times TFA = R \times TRA$, how many pounds of pull must the deltoid exert to flex the humerus?

$TFA = 2$ in
$R = 20$ lb   *ANSWER:*
$TRA = 15$ in

2. **Situation B.** The deltoid again is flexing the humerus, but the hands contain a 50-lb dumbbell. The resistance has increased and length of the true resistance arm also has increased. How many pounds of pull must the deltoid now exert to flex the humerus?

$TFA = 2$ in
$R = 70$ lb   *ANSWER:*
$TRA = 36$ in

3. Questions.

   a. What two factors cause the increase in force required in Situation B?

   b. Is the amount of force calculated in activities 1 and 2 sufficient to move the joint?

TORQUE

CONCEPT 51: Forces Acting on Joints can be Divided into Two Components: Rotatory and Nonrotatory

INFORMATION:

1. The force provided by a contracting muscle or by gravity (resistance) is subdivided into two components: rotatory and nonrotatory.

2. The only time the force of a muscle and the force of gravity are not subdivided is when the angle of pull is 90 degrees.

3. Whenever the angle of pull of a muscle differs from 90 degrees, much of the force produced may go into the undesired action (nonrotatory component) of stabilizing the joint and the rest to the desired action of producing torque (rotatory component).

4. Whenever the angle of pull of gravity (resistance) differs from 90 degrees, much of the force produced may go into the undesired action (nonrotatory component) of dislocating the joint and the rest to the desired action of producing torque (rotatory component).

RATIONALE:

For example, when a resistance causes movement at a joint, as in the case of a heavy weight causing the forearm to move from elbow flexion to elbow extension, not all of the force of the pull of gravity on the resistance produces elbow extension. The pull of gravity can also be subdivided into a rotatory and nonrotatory component. The former component pulls the forearm into a position of complete extension. The latter component serves to bring about instability (dislocation) of the joint.

The following diagram summarizes the factors involved in the production of torque at the joints.

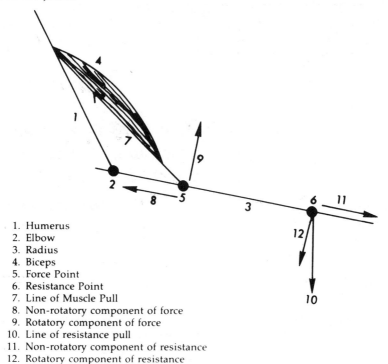

1. Humerus
2. Elbow
3. Radius
4. Biceps
5. Force Point
6. Resistance Point
7. Line of Muscle Pull
8. Non-rotatory component of force
9. Rotatory component of force
10. Line of resistance pull
11. Non-rotatory component of resistance
12. Rotatory component of resistance

ACTIVITIES:

1. Complete the following table:

	I	II	III	IV	V	VI
	F	FA	Product $F \times FA$ (Ft-lb)	TFA	Product $F \times TFA$ *	Difference $III - V^2$ **
A	100	1"	8.33	½"	4.17 ft-lb	4.16
B	100	2"		1"		
C	200	2"		½"		
D	150	1"		1"		
E	50	2"		¼"		

*Torque available to cause motion
**Force used for some other purpose.

128

2. Questions regarding activity 1.

    a. What is another term for the torque represented in column V?

    b. What term applies to the force represented in column VI?

    c. What must be the angle of pull of the biceps on the radius in situation D in the chart above?

TORQUE

CONCEPT 52: Nonrotatory Components of Muscle Force (Pull) and Resistance Yield "Undesired" Actions

INFORMATION:

1. Previous concepts explain that a force can be subdivided into components. In human mechanics, the force produced by a contracting muscle and by resistance (gravity) can be subdivided into **rotatory** and **nonrotatory components**.

2. The purpose of the rotatory components of muscle pull and of the resistance is to produce motion at the joints.

3. The nonrotatory component of resistance attempts to dislocate the joint.

4. The nonrotatory component of muscle pull stabilizes the joint.

RATIONALE:

A person who hangs by the hands with the arms extended from a chin-up bar for any length of time feels pain in the elbows. The ulna and the humerus feel as if they are being pulled apart. The explanation lies in the fact that all of the force of gravity is nonrotatory and is attempting to dislocate the elbow joint.

When a person attempts to flex the elbow while the hands hold a heavy weight, the task is difficult because the force of the elbow flexors is subdivided. The nonrotatory component is used to stabilize the elbow joint against the effect of the nonrotatory component of gravity which seeks to dislocate the elbow.

Stability of many of the joints of the human body is as much a result of muscle pull as it is a result of ligamentous support. Specifically, it is the nonrotatory component of muscle pull that contributes to joint stability.

131

ACTIVITIES:

1. Refer to activity 1 in Concept 51.

    a. What is the purpose of the force listed in column VI?

    b. If activity 1 calculated the effects of gravity rather than muscle pull, what would be the purpose of the torque listed in column VI?

2. Discuss the differences between spurt muscles and shunt muscles.

    a. Do spurt muscles or shunt muscles have the greater nonrotatory component of force?

    b. Why are spurt muscles capable of moving joints with greater speed than shunt muscles?

TORQUE

CONCEPT 53: The Angle of Muscle Pull Changes as Joint Movement Occurs

INFORMATION:

1. The *angle of pull* of a muscle is formed between the plane of the bone and the *line of pull of the muscle*, which lies along the long axis of the muscle.

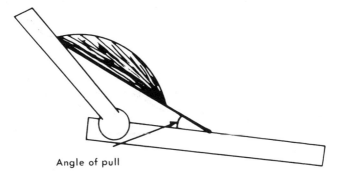

Angle of pull

2. When the angle of pull of a muscle on a bone is 90 degrees, all of the force of the contracting muscle is rotatory and is useful in producing torque at the joint. At any other angle a portion of the muscle pull is nonrotatory. As the angle deviates from 90 degrees (in either direction), the rotatory component decreases and the nonrotatory component increases. At an angle of pull of 45 degrees, the force is divided equally between the two components.
3. Movements of bones which articulate at joints produce changes in the angle of pull of the muscles producing the movement.

RATIONALE:

When motion occurs at a joint, the bones which articulate to form that joint change their relative positions. As the bones travel through their allotted range of motion, the angle between these bones either increases or decreases in magnitude.

133

Since the muscle(s) responsible for movement at the joint insert(s) into one of the articulating bones, any change in joint angle can result in a change in the angle of muscle pull.

ACTIVITIES:

1. Given: A Bicipital groove of humerus
   B Elbow joint
   C Distal attachment of biceps on radius; angle ABC is the angle of elbow flexion. Angle ACB is the angle of pull of biceps.

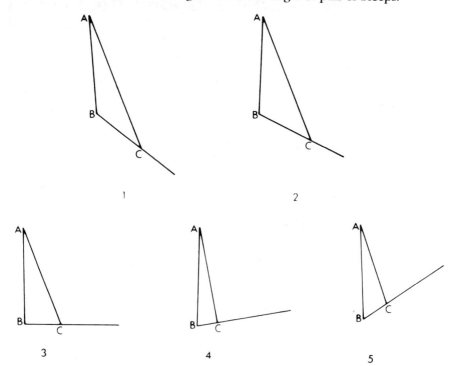

Use a protractor to measure the angle of elbow flexion (ABC) and angle of muscle pull (ACB). Complete the following table.

POSITION	ANGLE OF FLEXION	ANGLE OF PULL OF BICEPS
	Angle ABC	*Angle ACB*
1		
2		
3		
4		
5		

2. Questions regarding activity 1.

    a. Which position provides the greatest rotatory component of muscular force?

    b. Which position provides the greatest nonrotatory component of muscular force?

    c. Which position most closely approximates the position in which the available muscle force is divided equally between rotatory and non-rotatory components?

TORQUE

CONCEPT 54: The Angle of Pull of a Muscle Subdivides the Total Force of a Contracting Muscle into Two Components

INFORMATION:

1. The angle of pull of a contracting muscle subdivides the total force produced by that muscle into rotatory and nonrotatory components.
2. The rotatory component produces motion at the joint spanned by that contracting muscle.
3. The nonrotatory component stabilizes the joint against the strain of the resistance.

RATIONALE:

When the angle of pull of a muscle on a bone is zero degrees, all of the force of that contracting muscle is in the nonrotatory component and is used to stabilize the joint. As the angle of pull increases toward 90 degrees, force is taken from the nonrotatory component and is added to the rotatory component. At an angle of pull of 90 degrees, all of the force of the contracting muscle is in the rotatory component. This is when the muscle enjoys its greatest mechanical advantage. As the angle of pull increases beyond 90 degrees, force is taken from the rotatory and added to the nonrotatory component (see diagram below).

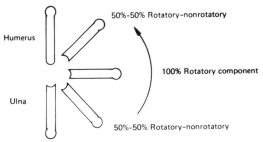

Theoretical expression of the two force components.

137

ACTIVITIES:

1. Complete the following table.

ANGLE OF PULL	PER CENT OF WORK IN ROTATORY COMPONENT	PER CENT OF WORK IN NONROTATORY COMPONENT
0°	0	100
30°		
45°		
60°		
90°	100	0
120°		

Name _____

Section _____

TORQUE

CONCEPT 55: The Human Body is Mechanically Inefficient With Respect to Force Production

INFORMATION:

1. In mechanical terms, efficiency is expressed as the ratio of work output divided by work input (energy expended). The per cent of efficiency is found by multiplying this decimal by 100. An inefficient machine is one which yields a low return of useful work in relation to the energy expended.

2. A third-class lever is an inefficient piece of machinery. A loss of force occurs when third-class levers are used. This is because the true force arm in a third-class lever is shorter than the true resistance arm.

3. When the angle of pull of a muscle is small, most of the force produced by the muscle is nonrotatory and is not useful in producing motion at the involved joint.

RATIONALE:

The human body is mechanically inefficient with respect to force production because most of the joints in the body act as third-class levers with the force point close to the axis of motion. The result is a very short force arm in comparison to the length of the resistance arm. The muscles must generate great amounts of pull in order to move relatively light resistances. However, the human is mechanically efficient when speed and range of movement are desired.

The mechanical inefficiency of the body is compounded by the small angle of pull of the muscle on the bone. Only when the angle of pull is 90 degrees is the total pull of the muscle effective in moving the bone. Seldom does the angle of pull of muscle approach 90 degrees. A nonrotatory component of force is usually present and only a portion of the pull of the muscle is useful in providing motion at the joint.

ACTIVITIES:

1. Torque through elbow flexion and extension is represented in the following diagram. To simplify matters, only the biceps muscle will be considered. Let us assume that a weight of 50 pounds in the hand increases the total weight of the forearm to 55 pounds. The angle of pull of the biceps at this point in the range of motion is 45 degrees. (Use a ruler to aid in answering the following questions.)

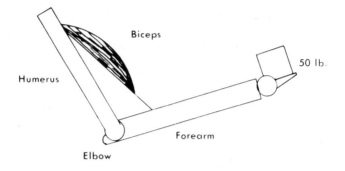

    a. What is the length of the force arm?

    b. What is the length of the true force arm?

    c. What is the length of the resistance arm?

    d. What is the length of the true resistance arm?

    e. How many foot-pounds of torque are exerted by the resistance?

    f. What force produced the torque in question e?

    g. To maintain the resistance in its present position, how many pounds of force must the biceps produce ($F \times TFA = R \times TRA$)?

h. Explain the answers to question g in terms of angle of muscle pull.

i. Which class of lever is in effect at the elbow?

j. Why is there a loss of force in this class of lever?

k. What two reasons for the mechanical inefficiency of the human machinery are illustrated by activity 1?

    i.

    ii.

TORQUE

CONCEPT 56: The Behavior of Levers Can be Explained in Terms of Moment of Force and Moment of Inertia

INFORMATION:

1. Useful concepts in body mechanics are those of **moment of force** and **moment of inertia**.
2. The moment of force is the product of the amount of force multiplied by the perpendicular distance from the axis of motion (joint) to the distal end of the involved body part (lever). (Note: $F \times TFA$.)
3. Because a motor act frequently involves the action of more than one joint, several moments of force can be involved in a skill such as batting.
4. The moment of inertia is the product of the amount of resistance multiplied by the perpendicular distance from the distal end of the lever to the axis of motion. It involves the distribution of mass. (Note: $I \times \Sigma mr^2$) where m = mass and r = radius.
5. The concepts of moment of force and moment of inertia are "two-way street" concepts.

RATIONALE:

The moment of force is another method of illustrating the behavior of levers. Muscles apply their force on a bony segment (lever) at a point near the joint and the lever begins to move. The distal end of the moving segment develops velocity. The longer the bony segment, the greater its velocity. Therefore, the longer the distance involved in a moment of force, the greater the linear velocity at the distal end.

The concept of moment of inertia is useful in explaining why certain resistances are difficult to overcome. This is especially true when the resistance is encountered at the end of a bony segment. An example would be lifting a light resistance on the end of a long pole. The light resistance is transmitted a long distance to reach the glenohumeral joint. The task would be much easier if a shorter lever (arm plus shorter pole) were employed because the distance involved in the moment of inertia would be shortened by withdrawing the mass closer to the axis of rotation.

Moment of inertia is significant in angular movement of the total body, e.g., somersaults or twists, or in specific body parts. Gathering the body or object's mass parts closer to the center of rotation increases the capability of body or body part to rotate faster. Thus if one *shortens* the moment of inertia, there will be a corresponding *increase* in angular velocity, a very important concept in several sport activities. Thus, in rotatory inertia, the concern is with the distribution of mass parts and not so much with the total mass.

ACTIVITIES:

1. The stick figure represents a bowler. Draw the moments of force from the following axes of motion: right hip, vertebral column, and glenohumeral joint (flexion).

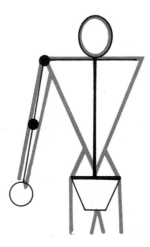

2. The following figures represent different patterns of throwing a baseball. Draw the moments of force for vertebral column rotation. (Note: The axis of rotation can be extended upward or downward.)

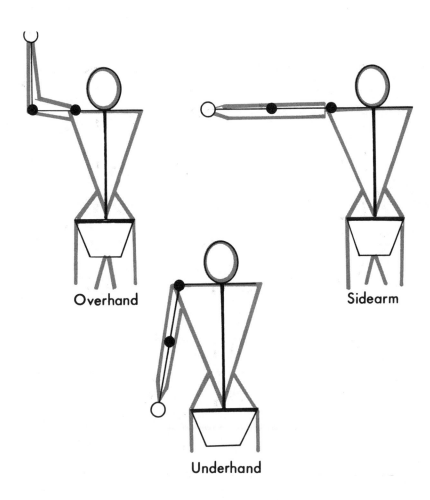

Overhand

Sidearm

Underhand

TORQUE

CONCEPT 57: Reducing the Length of a Moment of Inertia Produces More Efficient Joint Movements

INFORMATION:

1. Resistance, especially that produced by the pull of gravity, is capable of causing motion at joints.
2. A resistance is easier to move when it is located at the distal end of a shorter lever.

RATIONALE:

A person who wishes to lift a heavy object moves the body as close as possible to that object, thus decreasing the moment of inertia from the object to the joints providing the lifting motion. The downward pull of the resistance is transmitted across a shorter distance to the involved joints. The result is decreased downward torque. The lifting muscles must produce less force to overcome this decreased downward torque.

ACTIVITIES:

1. Why is it easier to lift a heavy barbell by positioning yourself close to it?

2. A person wishes to raise a 10-pound dumbbell by abducting the glenohumeral joint. In the first attempt, the elbow is extended so that the moment of inertia is 3 feet. In the second attempt, the elbow is flexed, resulting in a moment of inertia of 1.5 feet. What is the downward torque to be overcome by the deltoid in:

   a. the first trial: _____ foot-pounds

   b. the second trial: _____ foot-pounds

MOTION

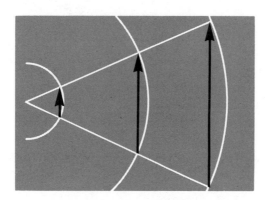

Concept 58:
The human body exhibits two types of motion: translatory (linear) and angular.

Concept 59:
Human locomotion is translatory motion resulting from angular motion at the force-producing joints.

Concept 60:
A joint exhibits angular motion, while the distal end of a limb may exhibit angular and/or linear motion.

Concept 61:
A greater linear velocity exists at the distal end of a longer lever.

Concept 62:
Walking and running demonstrate the alternating action of the upper and lower limbs.

Concept 63:
Many motor activities involve the principle of continuity of motion.

MOTION

CONCEPT 58: The Human Body Exhibits Two Types of Motion: Translatory (Linear)and Angular

INFORMATION:

1. **Motion** is defined as a change of position.
2. **Translatory motion** occurs when the body is removed from one location to another.
3. Translatory motion, commonly called linear motion, occurs in two forms. **Rectilinear motion** refers to the body moving in a straight line and **curvilinear motion** refers to the body following a curved, but not necessarily circular, path or moving around an axis that is not within the mass of the object (earth orbiting around the sun).
4. The second form of motion, *angular*, occurs when a body or object rotates around a fixed axis that is within the mass of the object (earth revolving around its axis). If the object is a lever, the distal end describes an arc or a complete circle.

RATIONALE:

The human body is often in motion in a straight line. Examples include a base runner going from home plate to first base, a person water-skiing behind a boat which tows the skier in a straight path, or a child sliding down a slope. These illustrate the form of translatory motion called rectilinear.

Sometimes the body exhibits the form of translatory motion known as curvilinear. Examples include running around a curve on a quarter-mile track and a skier navigating the gates of a slalom course.

Seldom does the entire body exhibit angular motion. This occurs only when the body rotates around a fixed axis, as in the performance of a giant swing on the horizontal bar. A somersault dive incorporates both angular and translatory motion. The somersault depicts angular motion; whereas the path followed by the body mass as it descends to the water describes curvilinear motion. Angular motion occurs at the joints of the body when the distal end of the bony segment describes an arc as the proximal end rotates around a fixed axis, the joint.

ACTIVITIES:

Indicate with a check mark the type of motion occurring.

ACTION	RECTILINEAR	CURVILINEAR	ANGULAR
Earth orbiting the sun		✓	
Elbow flexion			
Running home from third			
Rounding a bend in track			
Free flight in ski jumping			
25-yard freestyle swim			
The immediate path of a thrown ball			
The twist in a dive			
The path of a diver			
A "hook" in bowling			

MOTION

CONCEPT 59: Human Locomotion is Translatory Motion Resulting From Angular Motion at the Force-Producing Joints

INFORMATION:

1. **Locomotion** occurs when the moving object produces the force necessary for its motion.

2. **Translatory motion** involves moving in a straight line or curved path.

3. **Angular motion** occurs around a fixed axis that is within the mass of the object.

RATIONALE:

The source of the force which results in human locomotion is muscular contraction. The muscles pull on the involved bones which, because of torque, pivot around a fixed axis called a joint. Specifically, during the production of power in the walk-run, certain muscles cause the hips to extend, the knees to extend, and the ankles to plantarflex. These joint actions are examples of angular motion with the joints serving as axes of motion and the distal end of the lever, the foot, describing an arc.

The net result is that the body as a whole progresses in a straight (rectilinear) or in a curved (curvilinear) path.

ACTIVITIES:

1. Complete the following table.

ACTION—RUNNING ALONG A STRAIGHT ROAD

Type of motion _____

Subtype of motion_____

Force contributing _____

Joint Movements include:
Hip rotation, hip extension, knee extension, and ankle plantar flexion

Type of motion _____

2. Complete the following table.

ACTION—RUNNING AROUND A CURVE

Type of motion _____

Subtype of motion_____

Force contributing _____

Joint Movements include:
Hip rotation, hip extension, knee extension, foot inversion and eversion, and ankle plantar flexion

Type of motion _____

(Note: In activity 2, additional levers were employed. These produce the force which changes the path of the total body from rectilinear to curvilinear motion.)

MOTION

CONCEPT 60: A Joint Exhibits Angular Motion, While the Distal End of a Limb May Exhibit Angular and/or Linear Motion

INFORMATION:

1. *Angular motion* occurs when a body segment rotates around a fixed axis. The distal end of such a segment describes an arc.

2. *Linear motion* is synonymous with translatory motion.

3. **Angular velocity** can be measured at the axis of rotation and is expressed in units of degrees per second.

4. **Linear velocity** can be measured at the distal end of a moving body segment and is expressed in units of feet per second.

RATIONALE:

When a limb such as an arm moves, the proximal end of the humerus rotates within the glenoid fossa. Such motion occurs around a fixed axis, a joint, and is angular. The hand at the distal end of the moving limb may or may not be traveling in an arc. In either case, it would have linear velocity. The hand moves a certain number of feet in a certain number of seconds and may exhibit linear (translatory) motion. This fact can be demonstrated when a ball is released from the hand of a moving limb. The released ball does not orbit around the human body as it would if it possessed angular motion. Instead, the ball leaves the hand in a straight line, because the restraining force no longer exists.

An implement such as racket or paddle held in the hand of the moving limb also possesses linear velocity. This becomes evident when the student observes the behavior of a ball struck by a paddle. The ball leaves the striking surface in a straight line because of the law of inertia.

ACTIVITIES:

1. The following questions refer to a swinging pendulum.

   a. What type of motion occurs around the axis of the pendulum?

   b. Is it possible to make certain measurements and to calculate the linear velocity at the distal end?

   c. If the distal end of the pendulum struck a ball, what type of motion would be imparted to the ball upon impact?

2. During soccer activities, how can it be demonstrated that the foot has linear motion?

MOTION

CONCEPT 61: A Greater Linear Velocity Exists at the Distal End of a Longer Lever

INFORMATION:

1. If the force moving the levers remains constant, there is a direct relationship between the length of a lever and the linear velocity at the distal end.

2. *Linear velocity* can be determined by dividing the distance the distal end of the lever travels by the time expired ($v = d/t$).

3. The greatest linear velocity on a lever in motion exists at the distal end.

4. All moving segments of the human body are levers.

5. An implement held in the hand lengthens the arm as a lever.

RATIONALE:

Linear motion occurs at any point distal to the axis on a moving lever. The further any point is located from the axis, the greater that point's linear velocity. The maximum linear velocity for a moving lever occurs at the distal end.

When a lever is lengthened and the force moving the lever remains constant, the distal end of that longer lever travels around the circumference of a larger circle per unit of time. Thus, the linear velocity of the distal end increases. The opposite result would occur if a lever were shortened.

This concept is employed in many motor skills. The golfer who wishes to generate great linear velocity at the club head often selects a club with a longer shaft. The tennis player at the net who does not need to generate great linear velocity at the racket face brings the elbow into the ribs, thus shortening the arm-racket unit as a lever.

The diagram below depicts the relationship between the linear velocity and the distal end of a lever, with the angular displacement remaining constant.

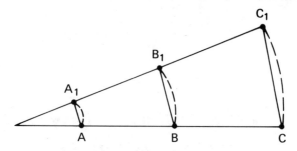

ACTIVITIES:

1. Given: An arm-racket unit traveling through the motion of a forehand stroke in tennis.

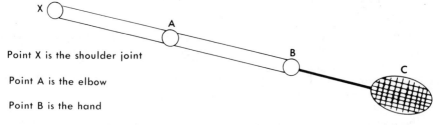

Point X is the shoulder joint

Point A is the elbow

Point B is the hand

Point C is the racquet face

    a. Which point, A, B, or C, has the least linear velocity? Why?

    b. Which point A, B, or C, has the greatest linear velocity? Why?

2. The following activities involve swinging a bat at a pitched softball.

    a. The batter swings a bat. The striking surface of the bat travels 36 feet in 3 seconds. What is the linear velocity of the striking surface?

    b. Using the same amount of force, the batter swings a bat of the same weight as in (a). The striking surface of the longer bat travels 42 feet in 3 seconds. What is the linear velocity of the striking surface of this longer bat?

    c. If the batter wished to swing a 32-inch bat with the same linear velocity as a 36-inch bat, what would he have to provide?

Name _____

Section _____

MOTION

CONCEPT 62: Walking and Running Demonstrate the Alternating Action of the Upper and Lower Limbs

INFORMATION:

1. In human locomotion, the leg which pushes backward against the earth is the propelling leg. The leg which is swinging forward through space is the recovery leg.
2. The moment of inertia for the recovery leg lies perpendicularly between the hip joint and the sole of the foot.
3. The arm opposite the recovery foot swings forward via glenohumeral joint flexion and is flexed at the elbow.
4. The moment of inertia for the arms lies perpendicularly between the glenohumeral joint and the finger tips.
5. In both walking and running, the knee of the recovery leg flexes as that leg swings forward via hip flexion.

RATIONALE:

During running, the recovery leg moves forward in order to place that foot on the surface in a position under the center of gravity of the body. To time this recovery act properly, the forward-swinging femur must have considerable angular velocity. Flexing the knee decreases the distance from the hip joint to the sole of the foot. The result is a decrease in the moment of inertia for hip flexion. Thus, an accompanying increase in the angular velocity for hip flexion is realized.

For purposes of body balance, flexion at the hip in the recovery leg should be accompanied by flexion at the shoulder of the opposite arm. The elbow of that opposite arm moves forward in a flexed position, resulting in a decreased moment of inertia for shoulder flexion. An increase in angular velocity occurs, and the arms are able to match the velocity of the rapidly cycling legs.

ACTIVITIES:

1. The figure below represents a person walking at a slow pace.

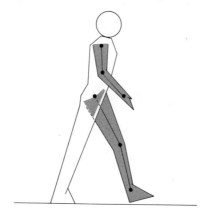

    a. What is the moment of inertia (in inches) for the left leg?

    b. What is the moment of inertia for the forward swinging opposite (right) arm?

2. The following figure represents the same person running.

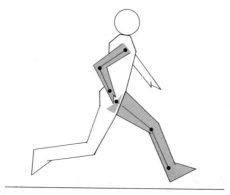

    a. What is the moment of inertia (in inches) for the left leg?

    b. What is the moment of inertia for the forward swinging opposite (right) arm?

3. Why does the shoulder in the first figure have less angular velocity than the shoulder in the second figure?

4. Why does the leg in the second figure have greater angular velocity than the leg in the first figure?

5. Why would a person with a stiff knee experience difficulty in recovering that leg when running?

MOTION

CONCEPT 63: Many Motor Activities Involve the Principle of Continuity of Motion

INFORMATION:

1. The principle of continuity of motion states that when a sequence of movements is employed in a motor skill, there should be no pause between them.
2. Motor activities demand that proper transfer of momentum be conducted so that desired outcomes are realized.
3. **Efficiency** involves a high ratio between energy input and work accomplished.

RATIONALE:

A single motor skill may involve movement at several joints. Several levers, therefore, contribute to the production of force. If a pause occurs between the contribution of any two levers in the chain, the force and momentum generated in any preceding levers are reduced. The result is a reduction of force for the entire motor skill and an imperfect performance. If a pause occurs between rotation of the vertebral column and movements of the humerus when one serves a tennis ball, some of the force produced by the vertebral column rotation is lost. The result is a weakly hit ball.

ACTIVITIES:

Write a brief explanation for each of the following mishaps.

  a. A batter interrupts the swing between body rotation and arm extension. The result is a weakly hit ground ball.

163

b. A pitcher's foot slips on the pitcher's plate. Hip rotation ceases; then, body rotation begins. The pitched ball hits the ground in front of home plate.

c. A basketball player pauses between hip extension and elbow extension during a free throw. The ball does not reach the front rim of the basket.

FRICTION

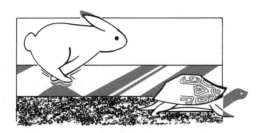

Concept 64:
A force that modifies motion is frictional force.

Concept 65:
In the absence of friction, horizontal movement is impossible.

Concept 66:
The coefficient of sliding friction is less than that of starting friction.

Concept 67:
The starting positions for many motor skills demand sufficient friction.

Concept 68:
Running in sand or mud is difficult.

Concept 69:
A second force that modifies motion is fluid force.

FRICTION

CONCEPT 64: A Force That Modifies Motion is Frictional Force

INFORMATION:

1. Frictional forces are defined as forces that press two surfaces together and oppose any motion.
2. The types of friction are: starting (static), moving (sliding), rolling, and stopping.
3. Factors that affect frictional forces are magnitude of force, materials at the interface, velocity of movement, and the irregularities of the surface.

RATIONALE:

Friction is resistance to motion created by contact between two surfaces. Starting (static) friction is greater than moving (sliding) friction; in fact, starting and stopping friction are synonymous and directly proportional to the amount of force holding an object against a surface. Because sliding friction is greater than rolling friction, it is advantageous to place an object on wheels.

Several factors affect friction. One is the weight of the object(s); usually the greater the force (weight), the greater the frictional forces—they are directly proportional to one another. Materials that interact and their irregularities can also affect friction. Friction is less when surfaces are smooth and hard; approximately the same despite the size of the surface areas in contact with one another; and relatively proportional to the size of the surface area when the surfaces are well lubricated.

ACTIVITIES:

1. Cite three examples of physical activity in which high frictional forces are important for enhancing performance.

    a.

b.

c.

2. Cite three examples of physical activity in which low frictional forces are important for enhancing performance.

   a.

   b.

   c.

FRICTION

CONCEPT 65: In the Absence of Friction, Horizontal Movement is Impossible

INFORMATION:

1. **Friction** is the resistance to motion created by contact between two surfaces.
2. **Starting friction** is synonymous with stopping friction and is directly proportional to the amount of force holding an object against a surface.
3. Friction is directly proportional to the weight of an object.
4. Formulas.

   a. To determine the *force (F) needed to start an object moving:*

   $F = kf$
   k = coefficient of starting friction
   f = force holding the object against the surface (usually the weight of the object)

   b. To determine the *coefficient of starting friction:*

   $$K = \frac{F}{f}$$
   F = force needed to start an object moving
   f = force holding the object against a surface

5. Maximal coefficient of friction equals unity (1.0).

RATIONALE:

During human locomotion and the performance of motor skills, friction is the "glue" between the surface of the foot and the supporting surface. Friction ensures that the supporting surface can push back against the foot with an equal and opposite reaction. The coefficient of friction is reduced when a person walks on an oily surface. When muscular force is applied to the foot, the foot slips backward. No equal and opposite reaction can occur from the surface and no forward progress can result.

A simple way to determine the coefficient of friction is to place one object (A) on a second (B) and slowly tilt the second until the first begins to slide downward. The tangent of the angle of the surface of the second object with the horizontal at the instant the first object begins to slide yields the coefficient of friction.

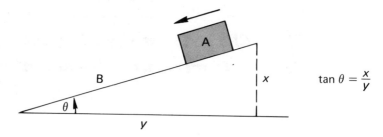

$$\tan \theta = \frac{x}{y}$$

ACTIVITIES:

1. An individual who is motionless on an icy surface weighs 200 pounds. A force of 100 pounds applied to the person will cause the person to move. What is the coefficient of starting friction of the icy surface?

2. The same individual is standing on a dry asphalt lot. The coefficient of friction for this surface is 1.00. How much force must be applied to the person before he or she will move?

FRICTION

CONCEPT 66: The Coefficient of Sliding Friction is Less Than That of Starting Friction

INFORMATION:

1. The **coefficient of friction** in a sliding object is always less than that of an object that is stopping.

2. It is easier for an object to continue to slide on surfaces with low coefficients of friction than it is for the object to stop.

3. **Sliding friction** is independent of the area in contact with the surface.

4. *Starting* and *stopping friction* are synonymous.

RATIONALE:

A person who begins to slide on ice continues to slide for a long distance if he or she remains on that ice. The coefficient of friction for the icy surface is low, so the person continues sliding.

An athlete who begins to slide while running on a wet field will slide for some distance. For this reason football players often employ "mud cleats" on wet fields. Such cleats are longer than ordinary cleats and increase the coefficient of friction between the shoe and the mud.

It is the increased coefficient of friction caused by the longer cleat that reduces the chances of sliding and increases the ability to stop once sliding begins.

Sliding friction is independent of the area of contact with a surface. If an athlete begins to slide on a surface, the size of the soles of the footwear makes no difference in the ability to stop. A wide-soled sneaker has no advantage over a narrow-soled sneaker.

ACTIVITIES:

1. A person runs along a wintry sidewalk and deliberately begins to slide on an icy spot. Why is stopping quickly so difficult?

2. During human locomotion, what component of force would have to be reduced to prevent the possibility of sliding on a slippery surface?

FRICTION

CONCEPT 67: The Starting Positions for Many Motor Skills Demand Sufficient Friction

INFORMATION:

1. The coefficient of starting friction depends upon the nature and condition of the contacting surfaces.
2. Friction is lessened by surfaces that are smooth, is not appreciably altered by dry surfaces, and is reduced on well-oiled surfaces.

RATIONALE:

Track sprinters wear spikes, football players have cleats on their shoes, and the top surface of a diving board is covered with an abrasive substance. All these methods affect the condition of contacting surfaces. Rough surfaces increase the coefficient of starting friction. Abrasive surfaces on diving boards present a very rough surface to compensate for the wet feet of the diver. Treads on sneakers also present a rough surface.

Spikes and cleats on footwear allow for considerable interlocking between the shoes and the surface. Interlocking increases the coefficient of starting friction.

ACTIVITIES:

1. Circle the letter of the examples which increase the coefficient of starting friction.

    a. Snowtread tires on automobiles
    b. Wax on a dance floor
    c. Abrasive surface on the starting block for swimming races
    d. Paint that contains sand and is applied to shower room floors
    e. Dancing slippers
    f. Spikes on golf shoes

g. Starting holes dug in a track

h. Soap on a shower room floor

2. What component of force or velocity is reduced when a decreased coefficient of starting friction exists for human locomotion?

FRICTION

CONCEPT 68: Running in Sand or Mud is Difficult

INFORMATION:

1. Friction is the "glue" between the surface and the foot which ensures that an opposite and equal reaction from the surface will occur.
2. Sand, mud, snow, ice, and other slippery surfaces have low coefficients of friction.

RATIONALE:

Sand, mud, snow, ice, and other slippery surfaces that have low coefficients of friction cannot push back against the foot with an equal and opposite reaction. Therefore, locomotion is inefficient.

When the foot strikes sand, some of the force of the foot is wasted in displacing the sand. Thus, less force is available to cause an equal and opposite reaction from the earth.

The same situation exists when a person runs in the mud. Some of the foot's force is wasted in displacing the mud. In addition, mud has a low coefficient of friction so the foot slips backward. A reduced equal and opposite reaction occurs, and no forward progress results. Ice and snow also have coefficients of friction.

ACTIVITIES:

1. Why does sand placed on an icy surface increase the ease of locomotion?

2. Why do some coaches encourage athletes to train by running on sandy terrain? Note: The force that displaces sand does not contribute to the desired result.

3. Explain in terms of starting friction the value of chains on tires during winter driving.

4. When walking on slippery surfaces, why does an individual shorten the stride? Note: When the foot strikes the surface, the foot is directly under the center of gravity of the body. This increases the vertical component of gravity. The force holding the foot against the slippery surface increases.

FRICTION

CONCEPT 69: A Second Force That Modifies Motion is Fluid Force

INFORMATION:

1. Fluid forces are of two types: air resistance or **aerodynamic force** and water resistance or **hydrodynamic force**.
2. Aerodynamic force is divided into two types of drag force: profile drag and skin friction. Both act opposite to the object's direction of movement.
3. Hydrodynamic force also has a drag force and is divided into three types: surface drag (skin friction), profile drag (form drag), and wave drag.

RATIONALE:

Aerodynamic drag forces depend to a large extent on the physical characteristics of the object being projected and upon the speed (velocity) of the air passing around the object. Generally, slow-moving air means the object also is moving slowly; thus, in this instance, skin friction is the important drag force. No significant turbulence is created, because the air flow is streamlined over the object.

However, during sport activities when objects travel at great speeds and turbulence develops, it is profile drag that becomes more important. If the object is large or exposes a large surface toward the direction of motion, a greater drag force will be created. Obviously objects that are streamlined or designed to create lift have less drag force and move more freely or with greater speed and distance through air. See the diagrams below.

Hydrodynamic drag forces include surface drag, profile drag, and wave drag. Surface drag appears to be the least important of the three types. It is caused by the

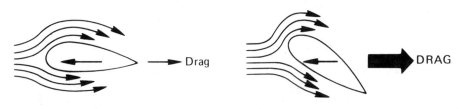

flow of water moving across the surface of the body. Usually the water passes freely backward across the body.

Profile drag is an important resistive force, because when an individual fails to streamline the body while "cutting" through the water drag increases. During the crawl stroke, the body should be nearly parallel to the surface of the water. If the lower body (legs) lies deeper in the water, a greater frontal surface will develop, and greater profile drag will occur.

Wave drag occurs when an object moves at the surface of the water and creates a lifting of the water or waves due to the interaction between the object and the surface of the fluid medium. The waves become larger as the speed of the swimmer increases. Wave drag is very noticeable in world-class freestyle swimmers and is directly proportional to the speed of the swimmer.

ACTIVITIES:

1. Diagram the air currents flowing around the following objects.

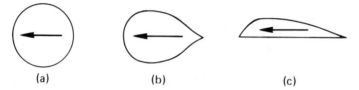

(a)   (b)   (c)

2. Which of the above objects has the greatest drag force, and which has the least?

   Greatest drag _____

   Least drag _____

3. Diagram the water currents flowing past the two swimmers. Which has greater drag?

Breast stroke   Free style

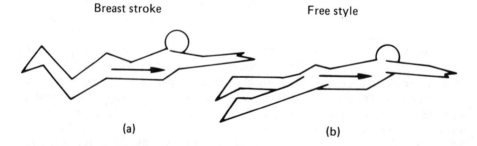

(a)   (b)

MOMENTUM

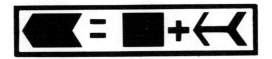

Concept 70:
Momentum is the product of the mass and velocity of an object.

Concept 71:
Changes in momentum usually occur because of changes in velocity rather than mass.

Concept 72:
Momentum at the end of a long lever is greater than at the end of a short lever.

Concept 73:
Motor activities incorporate the principle of transfer of momentum.

Concept 74:
Impulse is directly related to the concept of momentum.

Concept 75:
In motor activities in which the body becomes airborne, transfer of momentum must occur at the instant of takeoff.

Concept 76:
Many motor activities require that a performer reduce the momentum of an oncoming object.

Concept 77:
Many motor activities require that a performer provide momentum to an object.

MOMENTUM

CONCEPT 70: Momentum is the Product of the Mass and Velocity of an Object

INFORMATION:

1. Momentum is the amount of motion possessed by a moving object.

2. Formulas for momentum:

Linear momentum = mass × velocity ($M_o = mv$)

$$\text{Mass} = \frac{\text{Weight}}{\text{Force of gravity}} \quad \left(M = \frac{w}{32} \right)$$

$$\text{Linear velocity} = \frac{\text{Distance}}{\text{Time}} \quad \left(v = \frac{d}{t} \right)$$

RATIONALE:

The momentum of an object is the product of its mass multiplied by its velocity. Momentum may be changed by altering the mass of a moving object or its velocity. An object increases its momentum in a straight line when it maintains its mass and increases its velocity; an object increases its momentum in a straight line when it maintains its velocity and increases its mass.

The moving inertia of an object is proportional to its momentum. If two objects of equal mass travel at different velocities, the object possessing greater velocity is more difficult to stop. The same is true of two objects of unequal mass traveling with equal velocities; the heavier object is more difficult to stop.

ACTIVITIES:

1. Complete the following table by filling in the blank spaces concerning the momentum of four bowling balls.

BALL	WEIGHT	DISTANCE TRAVELED	TIME	MOMENTUM
A	10 lb	60 ft	6 sec	3.1
B	12 lb	60 ft	___	4.50
C	14 lb	60 ft	5 sec	___
D	16 lb	___	5 sec	6.00

2. Questions concerning activity 1.

   a. What are the two factors that determine the momentum of the bowling balls?

   b. Why is the momentum of ball B less than that of ball D?

   c. Which ball would strike the pins with the greatest impact?

MOMENTUM

CONCEPT 71: Changes in Momentum Usually Occur Because of Changes in Velocity Rather Than Mass

INFORMATION:

1. Momentum is directly proportional to mass and velocity. $M_o = mv$.
2. The following formula also is useful to solve momentum problems involving two colliding objects, provided one object comes to rest after the collision. The formula illustrates the law of conservation of momentum.

$$m_1 \times v_1 = m_2 \times v_2$$

3. The momentum of the first object equals the momentum of the second object.

RATIONALE:

Performers in motor activities seldom alter their own masses or the mass of an implement. To increase momentum, performers increase their own velocity or that of an implement such as a racket.

The linebacker who wishes to increase his momentum to stop a ball carrier simply increases his velocity. The tennis player who wishes to hit a hard smash swings the racket with greater velocity.

ACTIVITIES:

1. A 192-pound linebacker is running at a velocity of 10 feet per second. To what velocity must he accelerate to knock down a 224-pound fullback running at a velocity of 20 feet per second? ($m_1 \times v_1 = m_2 \times v_2$).

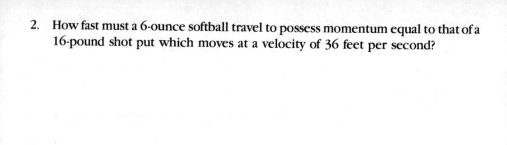

2. How fast must a 6-ounce softball travel to possess momentum equal to that of a 16-pound shot put which moves at a velocity of 36 feet per second?

MOMENTUM

CONCEPT 72: Momentum at the End of a Long Lever is Greater Than at the End of a Short Lever

INFORMATION:

1. The *linear velocity* at the distal end of a lever is directly proportional to its length (radius).

2. **Velocity** is a component of **momentum** ($M_o = mv$).

3. *Momentum* can be transferred from a moving lever to an external object.

4. It takes additional force to move a longer lever with the same *angular velocity* as a shorter lever.

5. Linear velocity equals angular velocity times radius.

RATIONALE:

   If it can be assumed that the angles of all clubheads are identical, then a golfer who makes good contact with a ball can hit the ball farther using a 5-iron than a 9-iron. The explanation lies in the additional length of the 5-iron, which acts as a lever in the golf stroke.

   Hitting with a 5-iron produces greater linear velocity than hitting with a 9-iron (provided the angular velocity is constant). The distal end of the 5-iron, therefore, possesses greater momentum which can be transferred to the ball at the moment of impact.

   The 9-iron, being a shorter lever, moves with a greater angular velocity than the 5-iron. In order to swing the 5-iron with angular velocity equal to that of the shorter iron, the golfer must apply additional force.

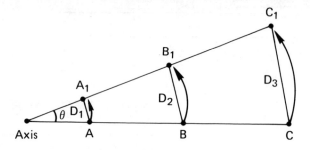

Lever A has the slowest linear velocity

Lever C has the fastest linear velocity

Relationship between linear velocity and length of the lever.

ACTIVITIES:

1. Batter A goes to home plate with a 35-inch bat. Batter B selects a 40-inch bat. The batters apply equal force when swinging the bats.

    a. Why could batter B hit the ball a greater distance when he made contact? Note: Angular velocity remains constant.

    b. Why would batter B probably have a high ratio of strikeouts to times at bat?

    c. Which batter is likely to possess the greater strength?

2. One reason that a driver will send a golf ball farther than a 3-iron is that it possesses greater mass. What is the other reason?

3. A long-legged man has thigh muscle strength equal to that of a short-legged man. Which man can kick a ball farther and why?

MOMENTUM

CONCEPT 73: Motor Activities Incorporate the Principle of Transfer of Momentum

INFORMATION:

1. The principle of transfer of momentum states that the human body is frequently put into motion by transferring momentum from a part of the body to the total body mass.
2. The same principle can apply to a ball that is put into motion by transfer of momentum from an implement.

RATIONALE:

In performing the standing long jump, the subject adds to the performance by flexing the arms at the glenohumeral joint at the moment of takeoff. Momentum is transferred from the forward swinging arms to the body. The same movement is used in some styles of the racing start in swimming. The momentum of a swinging golf club is transferred to a stationary golf ball. The velocity of the ball is increased from zero to great velocity.

The formula $m_1 \times v_1 = m_2 \times v_2$ is useful in solving transfer of momentum problems. If the mass and velocity of the body part or the implement are known, in addition to the mass of the body or the ball, then v_2, the velocity of the body or ball, can be calculated.

ACTIVITIES:

1. The arms of a standing long jumper weigh 24 pounds and move forward with a linear velocity of 15 feet per second at the moment of takeoff. The performer weighs 160 pounds. What portion of velocity at takeoff will be due to transfer of momentum from the arms?

2. The kicking leg of an athlete weighs 24 pounds and moves with a linear velocity of 50 feet per second at the moment of contact with a 3-pound ball. If transfer of momentum is perfect and the leg comes to rest after contact, what will be the velocity with which the ball leaves the foot?

Name _____

Section _____

MOMENTUM

CONCEPT 74: Impulse is Directly Related to the Concept of Momentum

INFORMATION:

1. **Impulse** is defined as the product of *force* applied over a period of *time*.
2. Impulse represents the change of momentum between bodies.
3. The greater the force and the longer the time the force is applied to an object, the greater the change in the momentum of the object.

RATIONALE:

Newton's second law of motion (see subsequent subsection); can be algebraically expressed as $F = ma$; where F = force, m = mass, and a = acceleration. Replacing acceleration with the following

$$\frac{V_f - V_i}{t} \quad or \quad \frac{v - u}{t}$$

the formula becomes:

$$F = \frac{m(v - u)}{t} \quad or \quad F = \frac{mv - mu}{t}$$

Then, rearranging the formula so it can be expressed as a function of force times time it becomes

$$Ft = mv - mv$$

Thus, the impulse of a force ($f \times t$) is equal to the change of momentum of an object ($mv - mu$) that is subsequently produced by the impulse.

It becomes obvious as the velocity of a given mass increases that either the force being applied to that object had to increase or its time of force application had to increase. Thus, the *impulse* had to increase as well. This is an excellent example of Newton's second law of acceleration. When a force is increased or the time of the force application is increased, the resultant change in momentum will be directly affected by the magnitude of the impulse.

It is important either to apply sufficient force or impart force for a sufficient time or both when performing such sport skills as shot putting, sprint starting, hammer throwing, baseball throwing, or bowling. The application of impulse is significant to the enhancement of sport performance.

ACTIVITIES:

1. Cite three examples of impulse use in sport skills where the performer is propelling an object in overhead action.

   a.

   b.

   c.

2. Cite three examples of impulse use in sport skills where the performer is propelling an object via striking.

   a.

   b.

   c.

Name _____

Section _____

MOMENTUM

CONCEPT 75: In Motor Activities in Which the Body Becomes Airborne, Transfer of Momentum Must Occur at the Instant of Takeoff

INFORMATION:

1. The body is often put into motion by transfer of momentum from a part of the body to the total body mass.
2. If transfer of momentum is attempted prior to takeoff, the momentum of the body part dissipates before the body leaves the surface.
3. If transfer of momentum is attempted after the body is airborne, the body is subject to Newton's third law.

RATIONALE:

In performing the standing long jump, the performer may flex the arms too soon. If so, the momentum built up in the forward moving arms dissipates during the lag period before the body leaves the surface. The result is a poor performance. Sometimes a performer may wait until being airborne to flex the arms. The individual is now subject to Newton's third law. As the arms swing forward and upward (action), the legs are forced downward and backward by reaction. The result is that the feet are placed in a disadvantageous landing position.

To contribute to performances, the transfer of momentum from arms to body must occur at the exact moment of takeoff.

ACTIVITIES:

Row I shows transfer of momentum occurring properly just prior to takeoff or contact in three motor activities.

Row II shows the same motion occurring after the performer leaves the surface in the same three motor activities. In row II, indicate by arrows how transfer of momentum will affect the airborne body.

Row I

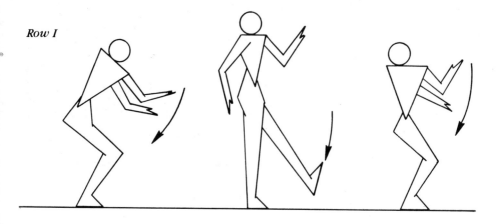

Row II

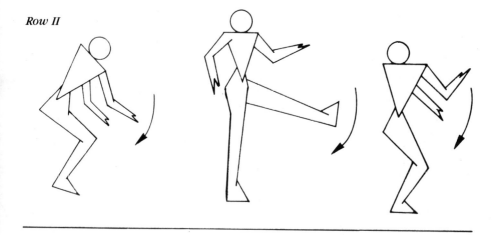

MOMENTUM

CONCEPT 76: Many Motor Activities Require That a Performer Reduce the Momentum of an Oncoming Object

INFORMATION:

1. Landing, one of the most fundamental skills performed in motor activities, demands proper execution of technique if the performer is to avoid injury. Skills in acrobatic stunts and combative games are examples.
2. Catching external objects can be difficult, because a premium is placed on an individual's motor and perceptual abilities.
3. Both landing and catching share similar mechanical applications, and one fundamental principle involved is the dissipation of energy.

RATIONALE:

When performing on hard surfaces, individuals may be aided in landing by using proper footwear, or, in the case of stunts and tumbling, by mats. The absorptive qualities of such equipment protect the body from injury. Some of the momentum of the body is dissipated when the sole of the footwear compacts against the mat.

Many mechanical factors are considered in the execution of catching techniques. The individual is asked to "give with the ball" to reduce its kinetic energy or is allowed to increase the absorbing surface by using a glove.

ACTIVITIES:

1. List four fundamental teaching principles for landing that should be given in the instruction of a gymnastic unit.

   a.

193

b.

c.

d.

2. Compare and contrast the mechanical principles that should be used in receiving the impetus of a baseball with those principles used in receiving the impetus of an offensive ball carrier in football.

   Baseball

   Football

MOMENTUM

CONCEPT 77: Many Motor Activities Require That a Performer Provide Momentum to an Object

INFORMATION:

1. Through the use of throwing and striking patterns, objects at rest or objects in motion can experience gains in velocity.
2. When the velocity of an object increases, its momentum also increases.
3. When you are throwing or striking an object for distance, a longer lever is more advantageous than a shorter lever.

RATIONALE:

An object at rest must be accelerated to be placed in motion. A golf ball on the tee has zero velocity, zero momentum. Its velocity is increased and momentum imparted when the ball is hit by the moving club head.

An object in motion may be accelerated when struck with an implement. A slow-pitched softball arrives at home plate with a given velocity. When hit by a swinging bat, the ball receives an increase in velocity and momentum.

Three throwing or striking patterns are commonly used in sport activities: the overhand, the sidearm, and the underhand. In all three, a longer lever system can produce a greater velocity at impact or release than can a shorter lever system.

ACTIVITIES:

1. List three sport skills in which an overarm pattern is used.

    a.

    b.

c.

2. List three sport skills, different from those in activity 1, in which a sidearm pattern is used.

    a.

    b.

    c.

3. List three sport skills other than those in activities 1 and 2 in which an underhand pattern is used.

    a.

    b.

    c.

NEWTON'S LAWS OF MOTION

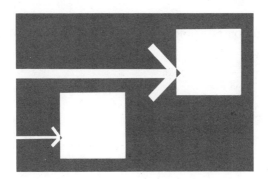

Concept 78:
A body continues in its state of rest or in uniform motion in a straight line, except when compelled by impressed forces to change that state.

Concept 79:
Inertia concerns bodies at rest and bodies in motion.

Concept 80:
Inertia is directly proportional to mass.

Concept 81:
A force is necessary to overcome inertia.

Concept 82:
The rate of change of momentum is proportional to the impressed force, and the actual change occurs in the direction in which the force acts.

Concept 83:
The greater the mass of an object, the greater the force needed for acceleration.

Concept 84:
If two forces of different magnitudes are applied to objects of equal mass, the greater force will provide greater acceleration.

Concept 85:

The law of acceleration aids our understanding of the law of free-falling bodies.

Concept 86:

For every action (force), there is always an equal and opposite reaction (force).

Concept 87:

The effect of a performer's action against the earth cannot be observed.

Concept 88:

The principle of action-reaction helps to identify the force that propels the human body during locomotion.

Concept 89:

The action-reaction principle is observable when a performer is airborne.

NEWTON'S FIRST LAW

CONCEPT 78: A Body Continues in its State of Rest or in Uniform Motion in a Straight Line, Except When Compelled by Impressed Forces to Change That State

INFORMATION:

1. Newton's first law of motion implies that everything in the universe is lazy.

2. The law implies an interrelationship between mass, force, and weight.

RATIONALE:

Many kinesiologists agree that Newton's first law has a variety of implications that are relevant to our understanding of human movement and sport performance. Some of these implications are that:

1. nothing starts or stops by itself;
2. a greater force is required to start a body in motion than is required to keep it moving;
3. everything in the universe is *lazy*, so lazy that a force is necessary to get it moving, when it then travels in a straight line; so lazy that once in motion, further force is needed to slow the object down, speed it up, or change its direction;
4. in terms of inertia, rest and uniform straight-line motion are manifestations of the same thing;
5. *inertia* is proportional to *mass*, the amount of the material of which an object is made; thus, in practice, the terms are interchangeable; and
6. less force is required to keep a body moving at a uniform rate of speed than is needed to stop the object or to change its speed.

Examples of how the first law can be applied to physical activity and sport include:

1. An athlete moving through space would continue to travel forever in a straight line were it not for fluid and frictional forces.
2. Anyone who attempts to stop a fast-moving object can testify that the object has a very strong tendency to continue moving.

Fundamentally, the law provides a definition for force and helps us understand the concept of mass and its relationship to inertia.

ACTIVITIES:

1. State three examples of the implications of Newton's first law for physical activity and sport.

    a.

    b.

    c.

2. Cite three examples of how Newton's first law can be applied to physical activity and sport.

    a.

    b.

    c.

NEWTON'S FIRST LAW

CONCEPT 79: Inertia Concerns Bodies at Rest and Bodies in Motion

INFORMATION:

1. Newton's first law states that an object tends to remain at rest or in uniform motion unless compelled by some outside force to change that state.
2. An object possesses *inertia* when at rest.
3. An object possesses *inertia* while in motion.

RATIONALE:

An object at rest possesses inertia. It will remain at rest until some force compels it to go into motion.

An object in motion possesses inertia. It will remain in motion in a straight line until some force compels it to change velocity, to change direction, or to stop.

ACTIVITIES:

Complete the following table for each action by placing an X in the proper column.

ACTION	RESTING INERTIA	MOVING INERTIA
Person at military attention	X	
Person dropping to a trampoline bed		
Shot put in mid-air		
Diver leaving springboard		
Sprinter at "take your mark!"		

ACTION	RESTING INERTIA	MOVING INERTIA
Baseball during the wind-up	————————	————————
Rolling ball	————————	————————
Ball contacting bowling pins	————————	————————
Ball leaving swinging bat	————————	————————
Wrestler who is pinned	————————	————————

NEWTON'S FIRST LAW

CONCEPT 80: *Inertia is Directly Proportional to Mass*

INFORMATION:

1. *Inertia* is the tendency of an object to remain at rest or in uniform motion in a straight line.

2. An object at rest and an object in motion possess inertia.

3. Inertia is directly proportional to the force causing the object to remain at rest or to move.

4. *Mass* is calculated by dividing an object's weight by 32, a constant figure for the pull of gravity.

5. Momentum is the quantity of motion possessed by a moving object, is calculated by multiplying the object's mass by its velocity, and is expressed as

$$(M_o = mv) \text{ with } \left(\text{velocity} = \frac{\text{distance}}{\text{time}} \right).$$

RATIONALE:

A heavy object that has a large amount of mass is subject to a greater pull by gravity and thus possesses greater inertia. The heavier mass requires a greater force to overcome its greater inertia and to put it into motion.

Because momentum = *mv, if velocities are equal,* a heavier mass possesses greater momentum and will require a greater force to change its velocity, to change its direction, or to cause it to stop.

ACTIVITIES:

1. Calculate the number of foot-pounds of work necessary to cause motion in the following resting subjects. ($W = F \times D$). Given: The coefficient of starting friction is 1.00.

OBJECT	WEIGHT	THE OBJECT MUST BE MOVED	WORK REQUIRED TO MOVE
A	100 lb	2 ft	_____
B	125 lb	3 ft	_____
C	150 lb	4 ft	_____
D	175 lb	5 ft	_____

2. Calculate the momentum of the following objects in motion. ($M_o = m \times v$).

$$\text{Mass} = \frac{\text{weight}}{32}$$

OBJECT	WEIGHT	VELOCITY	MOMENTUM
A	2000 lb	88 ft/sec	_____
B	2500 lb	66 ft/sec	_____
C	3000 lb	44 ft/sec	_____
D	4000 lb	33 ft/sec	_____

a. Which object would require the greatest force to cause a change in direction?

b. Which object would do the least damage upon collision?

c. Why does the heaviest object not possess the greatest momentum?

d. Why does the lightest object possess the greatest momentum?

NEWTON'S FIRST LAW

CONCEPT 81: A Force is Necessary to Overcome Inertia

INFORMATION:

1. A *force* may be defined as a push or pull.
2. A force is necessary to put an object in motion, change the rate of motion, change the direction of motion, or stop motion.
3. The force must exceed the inertia of the object at rest (mass) or the inertia of an object in motion (mv).

RATIONALE:

If a body is at rest, it will not go into motion unless a force is applied. That force must be sufficient to overcome the inertia of the object.

If a body is in motion, it will not change its velocity, change its direction of motion, or stop moving unless a force is applied. That force must be greater than the momentum possessed by the object in motion.

ACTIVITIES:

Complete the following table by identifying the force responsible for the listed changes in inertia.

CHANGE	FORCE RESPONSIBLE
Boy falls into swimming pool	Gravity
Girl propels a bowling ball	_____
Rolling ball hooks to right	_____
Bowling pin falls down	_____

CHANGE	FORCE RESPONSIBLE
Diver changes direction at end of hurdle	_____
Trampolinist contacting mat changes direction	_____
Sprinter accelerates	_____
Released shot put falls to earth	_____

NEWTON'S SECOND LAW

CONCEPT 82: The Rate of Change of Momentum is Proportional to the Impressed Force, and the Actual Change Occurs in the Direction in Which the Force Acts

INFORMATION:

1. Newton's second law of motion implies an interrelatedness among the quantities of force, mass, and acceleration.
2. Acceleration is directly proportional to the force causing the object to move and indirectly proportional to its mass.

RATIONALE:

According to several kinesiologists, Newton's second law of motion has a number of practical implications for physical activity and sport. Some of these implications are that:

1. greater force must be applied than that required to maintain a uniform speed for the body if it is to accelerate.
2. a greater force is needed for a heavy object than for a light one if it is to be accelerated faster than the lighter object.
3. when different magnitudes of forces are applied to two objects of equal mass, the greater force causes an acceleration in one of those objects.
4. a free-falling body is an example of this law because the force acting on the body is constant and causes a constant acceleration of 32.2 ft/sec/sec; and
5. an interrelationship exists between momentum (mass times velocity) and impulse (force times time) which can be demonstrated by the force equation ($F = m \times a$).

Examples of how the second law can be applied to physical activity and sport include:

1. A putter striking a golf ball moves the ball in the direction of the force applied to it, and the harder the ball is hit and the greater the force applied, the faster the ball moves.
2. A track runner is moving at great speed; to increase velocity near the end of the race, he/she must apply greater muscular effort to generate greater velocity or bring about an accelerated state.
3. A baseball pitcher uses a wind-up technique to increase the time it takes to apply force to the ball before releasing it, thereby involving the concept of impulse.

The second law actually gives us a better understanding of the behavior of objects since it explains the interrelationship between the cause of movement, the force and its effect, and the resultant acceleration.

ACTIVITIES:

1. State three examples of the implications of Newton's second law for physical activity and sport.

    a.

    b.

    c.

2. Cite three examples of how Newton's second law can be applied to physical activity and sport.

    a.

    b.

    c.

NEWTON'S SECOND LAW

CONCEPT 83: The Greater the Mass of an Object, the Greater the Force Needed for Acceleration

INFORMATION:

1. Newton's second law states that the **acceleration** achieved by a mass is directly proportional to the force applied and inversely proportional to mass.

2. A force is necessary to change the velocity of an object, either positively or negatively.

3. Acceleration is the rate of change of velocity. It may be expressed as positive acceleration or negative acceleration.

4. Acccleration is expressed algebraically as

$$\left(a = \frac{v_f - v_i}{t} \right)$$

    where a = acceleration, v_f = final velocity, v_i = initial velocity, and t = time (the length of the acceleration period). Acceleration is expressed in units of miles per hours per second or in feet per second per second.

5. Force is mass times acceleration ($F = ma$).

RATIONALE:

If two objects of differing masses are influenced by equal forces, the lighter mass will be accelerated to a higher velocity than the heavier mass. A greater force is needed to impart the same acceleration to the heavier object. Should equal forces influence a 10-pound object and a 20-pound object, the 10-pound object would receive twice the acceleration of the 20-pound object.

ACTIVITIES:

1. An automobile accelerates from 20 to 50 miles per hour in 5 seconds. What is its rate of acceleration?

2. A runner moving at a velocity of 10 feet per second increases velocity in a 2-second time interval to a rate of 20 feet per second. What is the rate of acceleration?

3. Complete the following table. (May solve by using a ratio.)

FORCE	MASS 1	V_i	V_f	MASS 2	v_i	v_f
100 lb	10 lb	10	20	20 lb	10	____
100 lb	____	10	20	50 lb	10	15
100 lb	10 lb	5	____	20 lb	5	7.5
100 lb	20 lb	5	10	____	5	6

NEWTON'S SECOND LAW

CONCEPT 84: If Two Forces of Different Magnitudes are Applied to Objects of Equal Mass, the Greater Force Will Provide Greater Acceleration

INFORMATION:

1. Newton's second law states that the *acceleration* achieved by a mass is directly proportional to the force applied and inversely proportional to the mass.
2. A force is necessary to cause *acceleration*. The greater the force applied to an object, the greater the resulting acceleration.

RATIONALE:

If two differing forces are exerted against objects of identical mass, the greater force will cause the greater acceleration. Should forces of 100 pounds and 200 pounds be exerted against two 10-pound objects, the 200-pound force would produce twice the acceleration of the 100-pound force.

ACTIVITIES:

Complete the following table. Use the information in problem 1 to solve problems 2 through 6.

FORCE	MASS	v_i	v_f
1. 100 lb	10 lb	10	20
2. 200 lb	10 lb	10	—

211

FORCE	MASS	v_i	v_f
3. 100 lb	20 lb	10	—
4. ___ lb	10 lb	20	80
5. 200 lb	10 lb	—	60

NEWTON'S SECOND LAW

CONCEPT 85: The Law of Acceleration Aids Our Understanding of the Law of Free-Falling Bodies

INFORMATION:

1. The law of acceleration can be expressed as mass divided by force.
2. To determine the distance an object travels in free fall, we use the following formula:

   $$D = \frac{1}{2} g t^2,$$

   where D = distance, g = force of gravity (use 32 feet), and t = time.
3. To determine the average velocity an object falls in a given period of time, we use the following formula:

   $$\overline{V} = \frac{V_o + V_f}{2},$$

   where $\overline{V}$ = average velocity, V_o = original velocity, and V_f = final velocity.

RATIONALE:

   Whenever an object becomes airborne, it is necessary for us to understand the use of the law of free-falling bodies. Sport skills, including gymnastic stunts, diving, and track and field necessitate the competitors' becoming airborne. Under normal circumstances, objects can be greatly affected by air resistance, but it is not significant when applied to individuals in regular sport events. Thus, for all practical purposes, air resistance can be discounted. The law is expressed algebraically as 32 feet per second per second; that is, under the influence of gravity, an object falls toward the earth at an accelerated rate of 32 feet every second per second it is airborne.

The distance an object or person falls is related to the square of the time during which the object is airborne. If the object is airborne for 2 seconds, there is a four-fold increase, for 3 seconds, a ninefold increase, and so forth. The distance can be determined by using the formula

$$D = \tfrac{1}{2} \, gt^2.$$

The average velocity between the initial measured point and the second measured point can be determined by ascertaining the initial velocity and final velocity after a given period of time, usually one second, of an object as it vertically descends. Average velocity is determined by using the formula

$$\overline{V} = \frac{V_o + V_f}{2}.$$

An example of an object falling during a period of 4 seconds.

DISTANCE

1. 1st second: $D = \tfrac{1}{2} \, 32 \times 1^2; D = 16 \times \ \ 1 = 16 \, \text{ft}$
2. 2nd second: $D = \tfrac{1}{2} \, 32 \times 2^2; D = 16 \times \ \ 4 = 64 \, \text{ft}$
3. 3rd second: $D = \tfrac{1}{2} \, 32 \times 3^2; D = 16 \times \ \ 9 = 144 \, \text{ft}$
4. 4th second: $D = \tfrac{1}{2} \, 32 \times 4^2; D = 16 \times 16 = 256 \, \text{ft}$

An example of how to determine the average velocity that an object falls from its first second to its second second, from the second second to the third second and so forth.

TIME	AVERAGE VELOCITY
1. 1st second: $\overline{V} = \dfrac{0 + 32 \text{ ft/sec}}{2}$	$= \ \ 16 \text{ ft/scc}$
2. 2nd second: $\overline{V} = \dfrac{32 \text{ ft} + 64 \text{ ft/sec}}{2}$	$= \ \ 48 \text{ ft/sec}$
3. 3rd second: $\overline{V} = \dfrac{64 + 96 \text{ ft/sec}}{2}$	$= \ \ 80 \text{ ft/sec}$
4. 4th second: $\overline{V} = \dfrac{96 \text{ ft} + 128 \text{ ft/sec}}{2}$	$= 112 \text{ ft/sec}$

On the following page is a graphic illustration of the relationship between the distance the object falls in free fall and the average velocity between seconds. Note: Not to scale.

DISTANCE	SECONDS	AVERAGE VELOCITY
0 ft	0	
		16 ft/sec
16 ft	1	
		48 ft/sec
64 ft	2	
		80 ft/sec
144 ft	3	
		112 ft/sec
256 ft	4	

ACTIVITIES:

1. Determine the distance an object falls when it has been airborne for a period of 10 seconds.

2. What is the final velocity of an object for the last 5 seconds of a 10-second fall?

NEWTON'S THIRD LAW

CONCEPT 86: For Every Action (Force), There is Always an Equal and Opposite Reaction (Force)

INFORMATION:

1. A force acting anywhere always has an equal force acting in the opposite direction.
2. Forces work in pairs opposing one another.
3. The initial force (action force) is opposed by a second force (reactive force).

RATIONALE:

The implications of Newton's third law of motion are numerous. Basically the third law assists us in understanding that:

1. in mechanical analysis, two opposing forces are equally significant and occur "simultaneously," although in human activity (motion), it is the human who is perceived as being the originator of the force (action);
2. when one object exerts a force upon a second object, the second body exerts an equal and opposite force upon the first;
3. opposing forces cancel one another out when they emanate from within the same body; in sport activities this law manifests itself more often as equal and opposite forces in two distinct bodies.

The following are examples of how the third law is manifested in sport activities:

1. A basketball player rebounding a ball lowers his/her center of gravity and prepares to jump vertically; the downward active force against the earth surface is equal to the upward reactive force from the earth propelling the player upward.
2. A swimmer pushes against the water (action force), and the reactive force pushing back is what propels the individual forward.

3. A hurdler thrusts the lead leg forward to go over the hurdle as the active force below the center of gravity causes the upper body to be moved forward in reaction above the center of gravity; in this way an extended leg and forward trunk lean position over the hurdle is created.

It should be pointed out that if an individual wishes to generate a rotating movement while airborne, the rotation has to be initiated from the earth; otherwise any action while the person is airborne will result in an equal and opposite reaction within the same object (the person) resulting in no rotation whatsoever.

ACTIVITIES:

1. State three examples of the implications of Newton's third law for physical activity and sport.

    a.

    b.

    c.

2. Cite three examples of how Newton's third law can be applied to physical activity and sport.

    a.

    b.

    c.

NEWTON'S THIRD LAW

CONCEPT 87: The Effect of a Performer's Action Against the Earth Cannot be Observed

INFORMATION:

1. Newton's third law states that every action produces an equal and opposite reaction.
2. A force exerted against the earth should cause the earth to move.

RATIONALE:

A performer standing on any fixed surface becomes a part of the mass of the earth. When such a performer exerts a force against the surface, we observe the action of the performer. However, we do not see the result of any reaction on the part of the earth. Because of its immense mass, the earth does not move any observable distance in response to the action of the performer.

A performer who stands on a tumbling mat flexes the trunk, which moves downward. According to Newton's third law, the legs would be expected to rise by equal and opposite action to meet the descending trunk. The legs do not move because the feet are in contact with the earth, which is too massive for one to move. The earth moves infinitesimally, but this motion is too slight to be seen.

ACTIVITIES:

1. In performing a vertical jump test, the subject flexes the hips and knees. The person then forcefully extends the hips and knees and plantarflexes the ankles. The body rises vertically above the surface.

   a. What is the observable action on the part of the subject?

b. What is the force that produces this action?

c. Why is there no observable reaction on the part of the earth?

2. In performing a tumbling stunt, why is it easier to gain height from the surface of a small trampoline than from the surface of the floor?

NEWTON'S THIRD LAW

CONCEPT 88: *The Principle of Action-Reaction Helps to Identify the Force That Propels the Human Body During Locomotion*

INFORMATION:

1. Newton's third law reveals than an equal and opposite reaction occurs as the result of an action.

2. During human locomotion, three lever systems produce forces that are exerted against the surface. These levers are the hip and knee, through extension, and the ankle, through plantar flexion.

3. A force can be subdivided into components.

RATIONALE:

During locomotion, the muscles which extend the hip and the knee and which plantarflex the ankle, produce a force which flows downward and backward and is transmitted to the earth through the foot of the propelling leg. This force is an action. For locomotion to occur, a reaction must flow back from the earth.

The reaction force provided by the earth flows upward and forward through the propelling leg and acts upon the center of gravity of the body. The upward component of reaction elevates the center of gravity and aids in keeping the body erect. The forward component of reaction propels the body horizontally across the surface and provides for forward progress during locomotion.

ACTIVITIES:

1. Place the letters below in the appropriate slots.

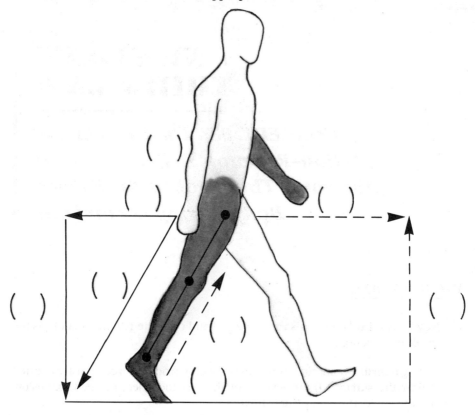

A. Propelling foot
B. Force generated by muscular contraction (action)
C. Vertical component of muscular force
D. Horizontal component of muscular force
E. Center of gravity of the body
F. Reaction force coming from earth (reaction)
G. Vertical component of reaction
H. Horizontal component of reaction

2. In the preceding drawing, the center of gravity of the body would be subject to the pull of gravity.

    a. Which letter identifies a reaction that prevents the center of gravity from falling?

    b. Which letter identifies a reaction that propels the center of gravity horizontally forward?

NEWTON'S THIRD LAW

CONCEPT 89: The Action-Reaction Principle is Observable When a Performer is Airborne

INFORMATION:

1. According to Newton's third law, every action of the human body should be accompanied by an equal and opposite reaction.
2. An action induced above the center of gravity of the body should produce a reaction below the center of gravity.
3. When a performer is in contact with the earth, there appears to be no opposite and equal reaction. The earth is too massive to be moved observably.

RATIONALE:

When a person is in mid-air and free from support, the body mass is obviously no longer affixed to the mass of the earth. During the airborne period, the law of action-reaction produces observable results. If the performer flexes the trunk (action), the thighs will rise toward the descending face (reaction).

ACTIVITIES:

1. An excellent way to demonstrate the principle of action-reaction is to stand on a stool which is capable of spin. Grab a baseball bat and try to perform the task of hitting an imaginary ball. What are the observable results? Explain.

2. A trampolinist, while airborne, extends the spine.

   a. Which way will the legs and feet move?

b. If one extends the spine while standing on the ground, why would the legs and feet not move?

3. A trampolinist, while airborne in a sitting pose, rotates the head and shoulders to the right.

   a. Which way will the legs move?

   b. If one performed this action while sitting on the ground, why would the legs not move?

PROJECTILES

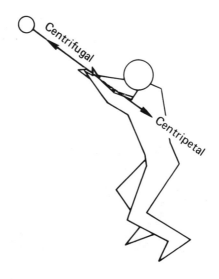

Concept 90:
A projectile's path is influenced by certain forces and the angle and height of projection.

Concept 91:
The trajectory of a projectile involves height, time, and distance.

Concept 92:
A projectile's path is influenced by impact and the effects of spin.

Name _____

Section _____

PROJECTILES

CONCEPT 90: A Projectile's Path is Influenced By Certain Forces and the Angle and Height of Projection

INFORMATION:

1. Several forces affect the path of a projectile: the propelling force, force of gravity, and drag (air resistance) force.
2. The projectile's flight time and distance are influenced by the angle of inclination and height of the projectile.

RATIONALE:

The human body and the objects it propels can be considered projectiles. When propelled vertically or horizontally in the air, an individual becomes a projectile whose predetermined path is influenced by forces, **angle of takeoff**, height reached, impact, and spin. These factors become observable when we deal specifically with inanimate objects such as baseballs, golf balls, racquetballs, discuses, and javelins—all objects in the sport world.

Probably the most significant force for any projectile is the so-called first force, the propelling force. With all things equal, the greater the propelling force, the farther the projectile will travel. Opposing this force, however, is the force of gravity and air resistance. Gravity's influence actually overcomes the upward component, and how rapidly it retards upward movement depends upon the weight or mass of the object, air resistance, and, of course, the propelling force. Air resistance has greater negative effect the faster the object is traveling, especially when the total amount of frontal surface area in the direction of movement increases. In addition, when the shape of the object is not aerodynamically designed, greater negative forces exist.

It should be understood that if the propelling force is constant, the angle at which the object is projected determines the height it reaches, assuming the beginning point where the object leaves the earth is the same as the terminating (landing) point. Also, if the rate of movement is the same for all objects, the height that the objects eventually reach determines the distance they travel because a relationship exists between the height and the flight time of an object.

In sporting events, it is necessary to project oneself or objects at varying angles to the earth's surface (ground). When vertical lift is important in events such as volleyball spiking, and basketball rebounding, then an angle of projection of nearly 90 degrees is necessary. In long jumping or hurdling, low projectile angles are significant because horizontal distance is paramount.

ACTIVITIES:

1. The optimal angle of projection is 45 degrees with all things being equal; however, for the following events would the angle be better if it were greater than or less than 45 degrees from the earth's surface (ground)?

EVENT	GREATER/LESSER THAN 45 DEGREES
Pole vaulting	_____
Outfielder's baseball throw	_____
Field goal kick	_____

2. Which force is prevalent in the following examples (gravity, propelling force, or wind resistance)?

EVENT	FORCE
Shuttlecock flight	_____
Baseball thrown from second to first base	_____
High jumper going over the bar	_____

PROJECTILE

CONCEPT 91: The Trajectory of a Projectile Involves Height, Time, and Distance

INFORMATION:

1. To determine vertical distance, use the formulas:

$$D_V = \tfrac{1}{2}\, gt^2 \qquad or \qquad Ht\,(\text{height}) = \frac{V^2}{2g}$$

   where g = gravity, t = and V = velocity.

2. To determine horizontal distance, use the formulas:

$$D_h = \overline{V} \times t \qquad or \qquad \overline{V} = \frac{v_o + v_f}{2}$$

   where D = horizontal distance, $\overline{V}$ = average velocity, t = time, v_o = original velocity, and v_f = final velocity.

3. To determine the velocity of an object, use the formula:

$$v^2 = 2gD_v$$

   where g = gravity and D_v = vertical distance.

4. To determine the time the object is vertically airborne, use the formula:

$$t = \sqrt{\frac{D_v}{.5g}}$$

   where D_v = vertical distance, g = gravity.

RATIONALE:

If a hurdler travels a distance of 12 feet and is airborne for a period of 1.5

seconds, what is the average velocity? Using the formula, $D_h = \overline{V} \times t$ and solving for $\overline{V}$, it becomes

$$\overline{V} = \frac{D_h}{t} .$$

Filling in the appropriate values, it becomes

$$\overline{V} = \frac{12}{1.5}$$

and the answer is *8 ft/sec.*

A high jumper reaches a height of 7 feet, 2 inches. What is average velocity and airborne time? Using the formula

$$t = \sqrt{\frac{D_v}{.5g}}$$

and filling in the appropriate values, we have

$$t = \sqrt{\frac{7.16 \text{ ft}}{16 \text{ ft/sec}}}$$

and the answer is *t = .67 seconds.* Using the formula $v^2 = 2gD_v$ and filling in the appropriate values, we have $v^2 = 32 \times 7.16$ ft and the answer is $v^2 = 458.24$ ft or $v = \sqrt{458.24}$ ft or *21.4 ft/sec.*

ACTIVITIES:

1. If a ball is thrown straight upward with a velocity of 18 feet per second, what would be its maximum height? (Assuming no air resistance.)

2. How far would a soccer ball travel along the ground if its velocity was 50 feet per second and it was airborne for 1.5 seconds? (Assuming no air resistance.)

PROJECTILES

CONCEPT 92: A Projectile's Path is Influenced by Impact and the Effects of Spin

INFORMATION:

1. A projectile's path is influenced by impact with a moving (striking) surface, by impact with an immovable surface, and by its elastic properties.
2. The effects of spin influence the path of a projectile.

RATIONALE:

Assuming it is possible to disregard the shapes or surfaces of two impacting surfaces, ie, the spin before and after or any elastic force, an object will come off or rebound from a surface at the same angle it approached the surface. See the diagram below.

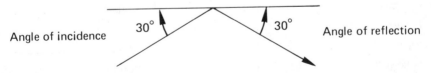

Angle of incidence   30°   30°   Angle of reflection

Therefore, the angle of incidence, that is, the angle at which the object approaches the contacting surface, is equal to the angle of reflection, the angle at which the object leaves the contacting surface.

When discussing impact, it is important to mention the concept of elasticity of objects. Elasticity varies in objects of differing substances and construction. A golf ball has great capacity to recoil from impact with a moving or immovable striking surface, while a shot put has very little. Some objects compress with ease and recoil with difficulty, while others compress with difficulty and recoil with ease. The capacity to recoil also is known as restitution. All objects possess a certain degree of restitution.

A simple technique to determine restitution of objects is to drop them, allow for free fall from a predetermined height, and note the height to which they rebound. Be sure the drop is vertical. Assuming you drop an object from a height of 4 feet and it rebounds to a height of 3 feet it can be roughly estimated as possessing a degree of restitution of .87. The degree of restitution is found by using the following equation:

$$e = \sqrt{\frac{\text{ht bounded}}{\text{ht dropped}}}$$

where e = degree of restitution.

Spin also plays an important role in projectiles. An object will follow an unstable flight path if it does not have spin, because spin assists in stabilizing an object in flight. Increasing the spin of an object can also cause it to curve, because of the unequal air pressures developed as it passes through a fluid medium. The direction of force by the striking object also plays an important role. For example, top spin occurs when you strike the object forward and upward; back spin when you strike the object forward and downward; right spin (clockwise) when you strike across right to left; and left spin (counterclockwise) when you strike across left to right.

When the spinning object strikes a horizontal surface, the following events occur. A top-spin object has a lower angle of rebound, a longer bounce and more roll; a back-spin object has a higher angle of rebound, a shorter bounce and less roll; and a side-spin object causes the object to bounce in the direction of the spin (right spin—right bounce, vice versa).

ACTIVITIES:

1. Determine the coefficient of restitution (e) for the following objects.

	HEIGHT DROPPED	HEIGHT BOUNCED	e
a. Baseball	4 ft	1 ft	_____
b. Golf ball	5 ft	3 ft	_____
c. Handball	7 ft	5 ft	_____
d. Super ball	6 ft	5 ft 6 in	_____
e. Volleyball	8 ft	4 ft 6 in	_____

2. Determine which way the ball will spin in the following diagrams.

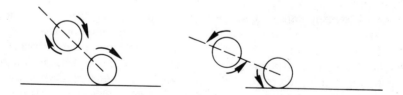

CENTER OF GRAVITY

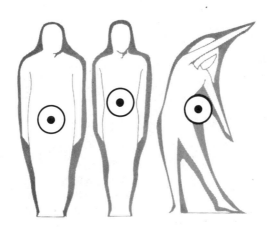

Concept 93:
Understanding the location of the center of gravity in the human body aids our understanding of movement.

Concept 94:
Each human being has a different specific location for his or her center of gravity.

Concept 95:
The location of the center of gravity in the body shifts when body parts move.

Concept 96:
The location of the center of gravity changes when external weights are added to the body.

CENTER OF GRAVITY

CONCEPT 93: Understanding the Location of the Center of Gravity in the Human Body Aids Our Understanding of Movement

INFORMATION:

1. The *center of gravity* of the human body is an imaginary point at the center of the body where the weight of the body is balanced.

2. The force of gravity pulls upon the center of gravity.

3. The center of gravity serves as an axis of rotation for twists and somersaults when the body is airborne.

RATIONALE:

Gravity exerts a constant pull upon the human body. This fact is obvious when the body is airborne. For purposes of mechanical analysis of motor skills, there is a reference point within the body where all of the body weight is centered. This reference point is known as the center of gravity. Its location may be plotted during the performance of motor activities.

The center of gravity is at the intersection of the three cardinal planes of the body. This point, however, is difficult to establish.

A rough estimate of the center of gravity in men is to locate it at 57 per cent of the standing height, measured from the feet. Because women tend to have a lower center of gravity than men, 55 per cent of their standing height is used. These figures refer to a person in the anatomical position. Detailed methods of determining the location of the center of gravity may be found in leading kinesiology texts (see Preface).

ACTIVITIES:

1. Draw the three body planes in the drawing below and pinpoint the center of gravity.

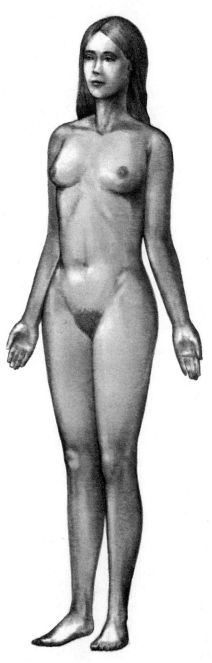

2. A male athlete stands 6 feet 2 inches tall. How far above his feet is his center of gravity?

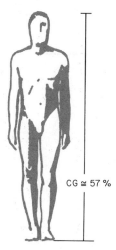

CG ≅ 57 %

3. A female athlete stands 5 feet 4 inches tall. How far above her feet is her center of gravity?

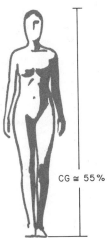

CG ≅ 55%

CENTER OF GRAVITY

CONCEPT 94: *Each Human Being has a Different Specific Location for His or Her Center of Gravity*

INFORMATION:

1. Most methods used to locate the center of gravity in humans provide close approximations and can be described as "points which represent the location of the center of gravity."
2. The center of gravity can be defined as a point about which all the parts of the body will balance.
3. Humans vary slightly in the dimensions and masses of their body parts.
4. Amputations and congenital deformities affect the location of the center of gravity.

RATIONALE:

Every human being varies slightly from others in the dimensions and weights of the body parts. These two factors influence the location of the center of gravity. Each individual has a different central point about which different size body parts should balance. Therefore, each individual possesses a distinct and separate location for his or her center of gravity.

ACTIVITIES:

Identify the approximate location of the center of gravity for each of the following figures. Drawing 1 is a standard model. The other drawings depict departures from that standard.

1.

2.

3.

4.

5.

6.

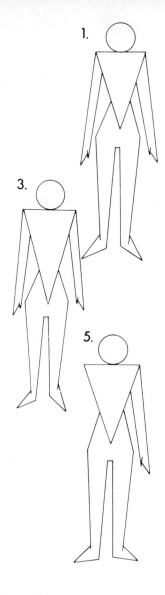
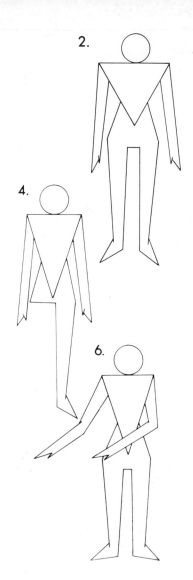

CENTER OF GRAVITY

CONCEPT 95: The Location of the Center of Gravity in the Body Shifts When Body Parts Move

INFORMATION:

1. Human movement is described from the anatomical position.
2. Methods are available to locate the center of gravity of a body while it is in the anatomical position.
3. Performers depart from the anatomical position when engaged in motor skills.

RATIONALE:

The previous two concepts are concerned with the location of the center of gravity of a body in the anatomical position. Seldom is the body in the anatomical position during the performance of motor skills. Body parts constantly shift their positions. Therefore, the points about which these body parts balance also shift. As a body part moves from the anatomical position, the location of the center of gravity shifts in the direction of that movement.

ACTIVITIES:

Identify the approximate location of the center of gravity in each of the following diagrams. Diagram 1 serves as a model. The other drawings depict postural changes from that model.

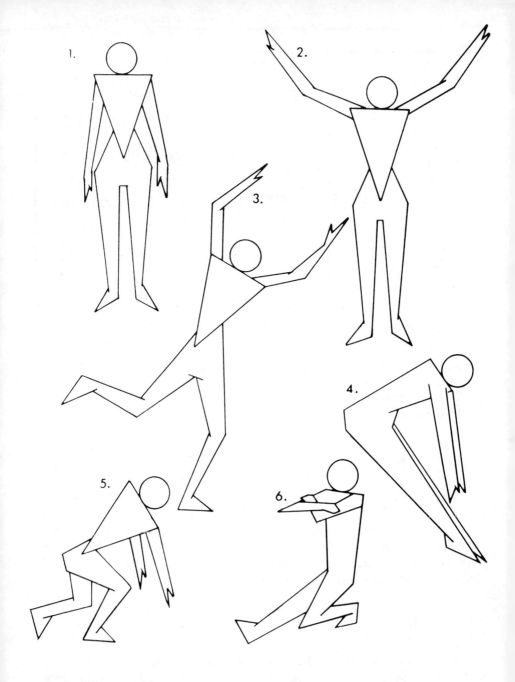

Name _____

Section _____

CENTER OF GRAVITY

CONCEPT 96: The Location of the Center of Gravity Changes When External Weights are Added to the Body

INFORMATION:

1. When external weights are added to a body part, distribution of the body's weight is altered.
2. If a person weighing 150 pounds lifts an object that weighs 50 pounds, the total weight becomes 200 pounds, and the center of gravity shifts in the direction of the 50-pound external weight.

RATIONALE:

Recalling that the center of gravity is the point about which all body segments balance, if an external weight is added to a body part, the weight of that body part changes. There must be a corresponding shift in the center of gravity to balance all body parts. The shift will be in the direction of the external weight. For example, external weights added to the ankles when running will cause a slight lowering of the center of gravity.

ACTIVITIES:

1. Which way does the center of gravity shift when a bucket of water is carried in the right hand? (The right hand is in the anatomical position.)

2. An athlete swings a 35-pound weight around his body as in a hammer throw. What is the effect upon the center of gravity?

3. In question 2, what is the effect upon the stability of the body and why?

4. In many countries people carry heavy boxes on top of their heads rather than on one shoulder. Why? (Answer in terms of maintaining stability in the frontal plane.)

STABILITY

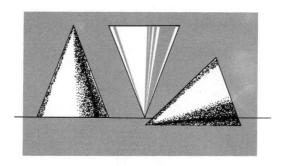

Concept 97:
The larger the base of support, the greater the stability.

Concept 98:
Raising or lowering the center of gravity within the base of support affects stability.

Concept 99:
Increasing the size of the base of support in the direction of an oncoming force increases stability.

Concept 100:
Stability and mobility are inversely related.

Concept 101:
Motor activities exist in which a performer desires to maintain stability.

STABILITY

CONCEPT 97: The Larger the Base of Support, the Greater the Stability

INFORMATION:

1. The **base of support** involves the points of contact with a supporting surface and the two-dimensional area between these points of contact.

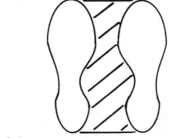

Left Foot

Right Foot

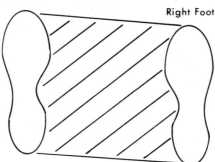

2. The **points of contact** are the body parts that touch the supporting surface. Examples are the hands, feet, knees, or any combination thereof, including the total body.
3. When the center of gravity of the body moves outside any margin of the base of support, stability is lost.

RATIONALE:

A wrestler on hands and knees is more stable than a wrestler who is standing. Since the margin of the base of support is further from the center of gravity in the first wrestler, it must be moved a greater distance to render this wrestler unstable. All other factors being equal, the larger the base of support, the greater the stability.

ACTIVITIES:

1. Shown below are the bases of support for a football player in a two-point, a three-point, and a four-point stance. The dot represents the center of gravity. Draw in the bases of support.

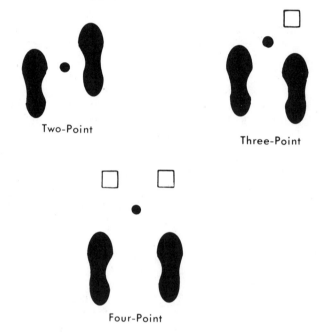

Two-Point

Three-Point

Four-Point

   a. Which drawing provides the largest base of support?

   b. In which drawing would the center of gravity have to be moved a greatest distance to go beyond any margin of the base of support?

2. In tumbling, why is the handstand a more difficult position to maintain than a head-and-hand stand?

3. An athlete suffers a knee injury. The doctor provides crutches so that the body weight will not be supported by the injured leg. How do crutches provide a useful by-product of increased total body stability.

4. For each of the stances below, give an example of a different but specific sport activity.

four-point position   _____

three-point position   _____

two-point position   _____

one-point position   _____

STABILITY

CONCEPT 98: Raising or Lowering the Center of Gravity Within the Base of Support Affects Stability

INFORMATION:

1. Raising the location of the center of gravity within the *base of support* reduces **stability**, since the center of gravity must be moved a lesser distance to cause a loss of balance.

2. Lowering the center of gravity within the base of support increases stability, since the center of gravity must be moved a greater distance to cause a loss of balance.

RATIONALE:

Most athletes realize they are more stable when they assume a semicrouched stance. The reason is that the athlete has lowered the center of gravity (hips) within the base of support.

Consider two people in separate canoes during windy weather. The first stands up and the canoe capsizes. The raised center of gravity in the man-canoe unit rendered it unstable. The second person lies prone in the canoe and does not capsize. The lowered center of gravity of the second canoe unit increased stability.

The higher the center of gravity, the less the body must tilt before the center of gravity goes beyond the margin of the base of support. The lower the center of gravity, the more the body must tilt before the center of gravity exceeds the base of support.

ACTIVITIES:

1. Consider the following drawings of a single block that has two possible centers of gravity, X and Y. In the drawing A, the block rests on its base; in drawing B, the block is tilted.

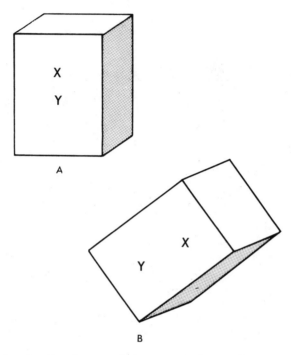

a. In drawing B, what would happen if Y were the center of gravity?

b. In drawing B, what would happen if X were the center of gravity?

c. Which position (X or Y) provides greater stability and why?

2. Why is it difficult to walk on stilts?

3. Why is it safer to kneel in a canoe than to sit on the seat?

STABILITY

CONCEPT 99: Increasing the Size of the Base of Support in the Direction of an Oncoming Force Increases Stability

INFORMATION:

1. The base of support can be extended in the direction of an oncoming force.

2. The center of gravity must be moved beyond any margin of the base of support to render a performer unstable.

3. If the center of gravity shifts toward the oncoming force while still within the base of support, stability is increased.

4. *Foot-pound* is defined as the amount of work accomplished when one pound of resistance is moved a distance of one foot.

RATIONALE:

A spotter is standing on the opposite side of a vaulting box from a springboard. Performers vault over the box. It is the duty of the spotter to prevent injury to any vaulter who crosses over the box out of control.

The spotter assumes a position with the feet spread in the **sagittal plane** facing the vaulters. The individual widens the base of support in the direction of the oncoming force (the vaulter). Stability is increased because a vaulter would have to move the center of gravity of the spotter a greater distance to push it beyond the rear margin of the spotter's base of support.

The spotter may further increase stability by leaning toward the vaulter. The spotter's center of gravity would now have to be pushed an even greater distance to render the person unstable. It is interesting to note that the spotter adopts a crouched stance which lowers the center of gravity. This factor provides additional stability.

ACTIVITIES:

1. Given: The coefficient of friction between the feet of a catcher and a surface is 1.00. The catcher does not rotate backward during collisions.

   a. A catcher blocking home plate has the center of gravity one foot from the rear margin of the base of support. The catcher weighs 200 pounds. How many foot-pounds of force are required to knock the catcher backwards?

      _____ foot-pounds

   b. Same as problem (a), except that the catcher spreads the feet toward the oncoming runner so that the center of gravity is 2 feet from the rear margin of the base of support.

      _____ foot-pounds

   c. Same as problem (b), except that the catcher leans toward the runner so that the center of gravity is now 3 feet from the rear margin of the base of support.

      _____ foot-pounds

2. What additional movement by the catcher will provide more stability?

STABILITY

CONCEPT 100: Stability and Mobility are Inversely Related

INFORMATION:

1. A mass that is stable lacks *mobility* and is moved with difficulty.
2. A "stable mass" can be moved only when acted upon by a force.
3. Two forces that frequently cause the human body to move are muscular contraction and gravity.
4. A mass that is mobile usually lacks *stability*.

RATIONALE:

The more stable a mass, the more difficult it is to move it. The more mobile a mass, the more easily it is moved, and the less stable it becomes. Thus, these two factors demonstrate their inverse relationship.

Walking illustrates this concept. Before moving, the subject is stable. Both feet are on the ground and the center of gravity is within the base of support. The person lacks mobility. In order to move, the subject exerts a force against the ground with one foot or leans to "fall" off balance. Thus, the center of gravity moves forward over the front foot, going beyond the front margin of the base of support. The subject lacks stability but is now mobile. The subject recovers the former rear foot and places it on the ground in front of the center of gravity to prevent falling off balance. Stability is momentarily re-established and progress is momentarily restricted.

ACTIVITIES:

Answer the following questions concerning the standing long jump.

1. In the preliminary position for this motor skill, does the body possess stability or mobility?

2. Before the performer's body can move, a force must propel the center of gravity beyond the front edge of the base of support. Identify this force.

3. At the height of the arc, what is the "visible" force affecting the center of gravity?

4. Upon landing, where is the center of gravity in reference to the base of support?

5. Why, upon landing, can the body no longer move to any extent?

STABILITY

CONCEPT 101: Motor Activities Exist in Which a Performer Desires to Maintain Stability

INFORMATION:

1. Many motor activities demand that a performer seek **static stability**, that is, remain motionless in one location. To accomplish this, the performer attempts to use all available sources, lower the center of gravity, widen the base of support, and so forth.
2. Other motor activities demand that a performer seek **dynamic stability**, that is, maintain balance (equilibrium) while constantly changing body position.

RATIONALE:

Many of our sport activities demand that a performer seek static stability. The wrestler in the down (defense) position does not wish to have balance destroyed by the up (offensive) wrestler. When weightlifting, a performer must have static stability when moving a heavy weight. In karate, throwing an opponent to the mat requires maximum stability.

Most of our motor activities prize stability while the performer is in constant motion, continually moving the base of support. An example might be the actions of a defensive basketball player attempting to stop an opponent from moving to a given position or a wrestler's fending off an attack by an opponent. The skill and grace of a performer on a balance beam illustrate stability while in motion.

ACTIVITIES:

1. A baseball catcher is attempting to tag a runner at home plate. The runner is about to collide with the catcher. Using previous information about

stability, list three adjustments the catcher can make to increase stability prior to collision.

    a.

    b.

    c.

2. A basketball player is guarding an opponent who has the basketball. The defensive player wishes to ensure body equilibrium while in constant motion. Three of the following statements indicate methods of meeting this goal. Circle the letter of the statements that depict desired goals.

    a. Take short steps to constantly re-establish the base of support.
    b. Make lunging movements to distract the player with the ball.
    c. Stand erect to occupy more defensive space.
    d. Lower the center of gravity within the constantly changing base of support.
    e. Keep the center of gravity in the middle of the base of support.

FOLLOW-THROUGH

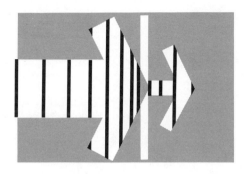

Concept 102:

Follow-through prevents a loss of linear velocity at the moment of impact or release.

Concept 103:

Follow-through prevents injuries caused by the abrupt stopping of a moving body part.

Concept 104:

Follow-through prevents the violation of certain playing rules.

Concept 105:

Follow-through provides time to perceive feedback information.

FOLLOW-THROUGH

CONCEPT 102: Follow-Through Prevents a Loss of Linear Velocity at the Moment of Impact or Release

INFORMATION:

1. The principle of summation of forces states that all body levers used to impart momentum to an object must make their contribution at the moment of impact or instant of release.

2. In many motor skills, objects are either struck by implements attached to the distal end of body levers or are released from the distal end of body levers.

3. The distal end of a body lever possesses linear velocity.

RATIONALE:

When a player bats a ball, the bat should achieve maximum linear velocity at the moment of impact with the ball. When the player throws a ball, the hand should achieve maximum linear velocity at the instant the ball is released. Note that both the bat and the ball are held at the distal end of the arm, a lever.

If the player were to allow the velocity of the bat or the hand containing a ball to decrease prior to impact or release, the result would be a weaker hit or a weaker throw.

Follow-through prevents a decrease in linear velocity at the moment of impact of bat on ball or at the instant of release of a thrown ball. By follow-through, the player maintains a steady contraction of the involved muscles until the motor act is completed.

261

ACTIVITIES:

1. In the process of throwing a baseball, a player ceases contraction of the triceps before elbow extension is completed and releases the ball prior to the completion of wrist flexion.

   a. How do these errors affect the flight of the ball?

   b. Why?

2. A tennis server reduces the force produced by the arm muscles just prior to impact of racket on ball.

   a. How does this error affect the flight of the ball?

   b. Why?

FOLLOW-THROUGH

CONCEPT 103: *Follow-Through Prevents Injuries Caused by the Abrupt Stopping of a Moving Body Part*

INFORMATION:

1. A moving body part has *momentum*. The abrupt reduction of momentum may cause injuries to muscles and/or joints.
2. Follow-through permits a gradual deceleration of body levers. The result is a gradual loss of momentum in these levers after impact or release has occurred.

RATIONALE:

When **agonist** muscles contract, body levers are set in motion and generate momentum. An abrupt cessation of the movement in these levers may result in too sudden a stopping of momentum and injury may occur in the moving body parts.

Follow-through permits a gradual decrease in momentum in these moving body parts.

ACTIVITIES:

1. If horizontal flexion of the glenohumeral joint is actively stopped by contraction of the posterior deltoid before the shot put leaves the hand, what may occur to the posterior deltoid muscles?

2. If a base runner attempts to slow down suddenly without sliding into a base, what may occur to the thigh muscles?

Name _____

Section _____

FOLLOW-THROUGH

CONCEPT 104: Follow-Through Prevents the Violation of Certain Playing Rules

INFORMATION:

1. Many competitive motor skills are governed by rules that legislate against stepping over certain boundary lines.
2. Follow-through allows for a controlled stopping of total body movement so that stability is re-established before boundary lines are violated.

RATIONALE:

A bowler delivering a ball strides toward a foul line. After release of the ball, if an attempt is made to stop the movement of all body parts simultaneously, the momentum may cause the bowler to cross the foul line. A violation would result. A similar example could be given for a shot-putter moving across the circle.

Follow-through allows for a gradual diminishing of momentum in the total body or its parts. Time is provided to re-establish a new base of support under the moving center of gravity. Total body stability is established before the body or one of its parts violates a foul line.

ACTIVITIES:

A basketball player at the free-throw line moves the arms at a linear velocity of 25 feet per second. The weight of the arms plus the basketball is 32 pounds.

    a.   What is the momentum of the arms?

b. Can the momentum of the arms be transferred to the body?

c. If the movement of the arms is stopped suddenly as the ball is released, how can the body be affected?

d. If the momentum of the arms gradually diminishes during follow-through, what will be the effect on the total body?

e. Was the reduction of momentum in question (d) caused by a reduction in mass or a reduction in velocity?

FOLLOW-THROUGH

CONCEPT 105: Follow-Through Provides Time to Perceive Feedback Information

INFORMATION:

1. Input concerning a given performance is fed back to the individual through the body's many receptors. This information (data) is used to aid the athlete in improving the next attempt at a motor skill.
2. **Feedback** permits an athlete to analyze a performance and to make corrections so that errors are not repeated.

RATIONALE:

At the completion of certain motor skills, follow-through provides a brief inactive period during which visual or kinesthetic feedback can be received and interpreted by the performer.

A tennis player whose initial serve is unsuccessful uses the brief interval during the follow-through to analyze the imperfect performance and to identify possible solutions.

A skillful free thrower in basketball knows, almost as soon as the ball leaves the hand, whether the attempt will be successful. During the period of follow-through, while the ball is traveling toward the basket, the player is provided with a brief interval to analyze the performance and identify possible errors.

ACTIVITIES:

1. Circle the letter of the activities which would present a period of follow-through during which an athlete could receive feedback and analyze the performance.

    a. A front somersault during a tumbling routine

b. A baseball pitch at which the batter did not swing
c. Missing the first of two free throws in basketball
d. A golf drive from the tee
e. A missed field goal in football
f. A left hand punch in a boxing match
g. A jump shot in basketball
h. Shooting an arrow in archery

2. A placekicker in football is instructed to keep his head down for a short period after the ball is kicked. Since he cannot see the ball in flight, what sense receptors provide him with feedback?

3. During the follow-through at the end of the delivery of a bowling ball, what analysis might be running through the mind of the bowler?

APPLICATION TO SPORT FORMS

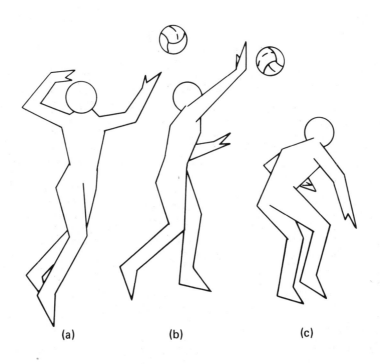

(a)   (b)   (c)

Concept 106:
Baseball/softball sliding uses the principle of receiving impetus.

Concept 107:
The jump shot employs Newton's third law of motion.

Concept 108:
Downhill skiing depends on the force of gravity.

Concept 109:
One foot must be in contact with the ground when a player kicks a football.

Concept 110:
The full golf swing uses an increased lever system to gain maximum linear velocity of the clubhead.

Concept 111:
Centrifugal force (inertia) and centripetal force must counterbalance one another during the performance of a giant swing on the horizontal bar.

Concept 112:
A floor routine during the free-exercise event uses a number of biomechanical concepts.

Concept 113:
A whirling figure skater uses changing moments of inertia to control angular velocity.

Concept 114:
There are some motor activities in which the performer wishes to lose stability in certain starting events.

Concept 115:
Effort that does not contribute to the desired result acts as resistance.

Concept 116:
Movement through the water is best achieved by the effective use of a swimmer's arms and legs.

Concept 117:
A diver can perform more somersaults in the tuck position, fewer in the pike position, and fewest in the layout position.

Concept 118:
Increasing the length of a moment of force produces stronger joint movements when striking (giving impetus to) a tennis ball.

Concept 119:
Follow-through places the body in a "ready position" to begin the next tennis skill.

Concept 120:
When the body is in free flight, no amount of maneuvering of body parts can alter the path of the center of gravity.

Concept 121:

Centrifugal force (inertia) and centripetal force must counterbalance one another during the hammer throw.

Concept 122:

Hurdlers must minimize their time in the air.

Concept 123:

The purpose of high jumping is to propel the center of gravity to a height sufficient for good performance.

Concept 124:

The forearm bump pass is an example of receiving impetus (momentum of an object).

Concept 125:

Spiking the ball is an example of giving impetus to an object.

Concept 126:

The use of levers is important to successful wrestling techniques.

BASEBALL/ SOFTBALL

CONCEPT 106: Baseball/Softball Sliding Uses the Principle of Receiving Impetus

INFORMATION:

1. Receiving impetus (momentum) of an object utilizes such principles as gradually decreasing the kinetic energy of the object, dissipating forces, increasing the time over which the object is slowed, and increasing frictional forces.
2. Although the primary purpose of sliding is to slow the forward momentum of a base runner, its practical use is to avoid being called "out" while stealing a base or while taking an extra base.

RATIONALE:

When a base runner is not concerned about being tagged out, sliding into a base is unnecessary. In fact, it is better for a runner to remain standing as it may be more important to round the base in anticipation of going to the next base. It is often necessary, however, to slide into a base, and understanding certain biomechanical principles should ensure proper execution of the slide.

Sliding can be accomplished in a number of ways. A base runner can use the hook, the pop-up, or the face-first slide. Depending upon the situation, each has advantages and disadvantages, and they employ similar biomechanical concepts. In each situation, the forward momentum of the runner must be slowed, then stopped at the base.

Whether using the hook or pop-up slide, the runner must lean away from the intended forward motion. This leaning away from the base during the approach induces backward rotation caused by the pull of gravity exerting its force behind the base of support, creating a backward horizontal eccentric thrust and by transfer of momentum as the person falls to the ground. The individual lifts the feet off the ground slightly and slides into the ground. In the hook-slide, much of the runner's surface area contacts the ground, increasing the frictional forces, and slowing the runner's forward progress. In the pop-up slide, there is less surface area in contact with the ground and the execution is directed straight at the base in order for the runner to come to a rapid standing position to proceed to the next base if necessary. The hook-slide technique is directed away from the base and there is no immediate concern to come to one's feet.

In the face-first slide, the same principles apply except that the runner imparts forward horizontal eccentric thrust (checking linear velocity) with the upper body rotating much faster than the legs, causing the runner to assume a prone position. Again, contact with the ground is made by a large surface area increasing frictional forces and slowing the runner down. Generally there is little concern about advancing to another base. Research suggests that the head-first slide might be the fastest sliding technique, possibly because forward horizontal eccentric thrust is a more rapid movement than backward horizontal eccentric thrust.

ACTIVITIES:

1. Ask five relatively proficient baseball/softball players to take part in a mini-research project. Select five individuals who possess the same or comparable speed between first and second base from a standing start and who are good at sliding. Ask each to begin their slides at a prescribed distance from second base. Give them at least two trials for each of the three types of slides. Use reaction time mats. The clock starts when they touch the first timing mat and stops when they touch the second timing mat located at second base. Explain your results.

Name _____

Section _____

BASKETBALL

CONCEPT 107: The Jump Shot Employs Newton's Third Law of Motion

INFORMATION:

1. For a player to execute a vertical jump maneuver, such as a basketball jump shot, an action force must be applied downward through the jumping surface with a resultant reactive force propelling the player upward.

2. The two forces must pass through the person's center of gravity or rotation will occur.

3. The mechanics used in the basketball jump shot are similar to those needed to spike a volleyball, rebound a basketball, or leap into the air to catch a baseball.

RATIONALE:

A number of biomechanical principles are used to prepare a basketball player to execute a jump shot; the most significant, however, is to give oneself vertical lift using Newton's third law of motion.

The jump shot is often used after a dribble or from a stopped position. To prepare for the execution of either technique, the player widens the base of support for increased stability, places the extensor muscles on stretch, and lowers the center of gravity—all for the explosive act. Next, the active force is applied directly downward through the player's center of gravity by the extensor muscles pushing against the floor. The reactive force is applied upward from the floor directly through the player's center of gravity to propel the person vertically into the air. All these actions are needed to obtain the necessary height for the jump shot.

If at any time the action-reaction forces of Newton's third law are imparted outside the person's center of gravity, a degree of rotation will occur, and some of the effective force for vertical lift will be "lost," resulting in less than the desired height.

275

ACTIVITIES:

1. Execute a number of jump shots using the following techniques: Jump while leaning forward, and jump while leaning backward. Explain what occurs.

2. Dribble the ball down the court and execute a number of jump shots. For the first few shots, dribble, slow down, lean forward, and jump. For the next few shots, dribble, slow down, lean backward, and jump. Explain what occurs for each technique.

Name _____

Section _____

DOWNHILL SKIING

CONCEPT 108: Downhill Skiing Depends on the Force of Gravity

INFORMATION:

1. Gravity exerts a constant downward pull on all objects. In skiing, the weight of the skier serves as the force which propels the skier down the hill.
2. The skier is affected by air resistance, which increases in magnitude as the velocity of the skier increases.

RATIONALE:

If a skier attempts a straight run directly down a hill, the only negative forces present to impede velocity are the frictional forces between the surfaces of the skis and the snow, and wind resistance. Generally, a rapid downhill run is only applicable in downhill racing. Most skiers traverse the slopes by making appropriate turns and stops to fully enjoy the exhilaration of the run.

A skier on top of a mountain has potential energy. This potential energy depends upon the weight of the person and the vertical distance between the top of the hill (mountain) and the level spot at the end of the run. These two factors directly influence the skier's velocity down the hill. Once underway, the skier possesses kinetic energy, the magnitude of which is similar to the person's potential energy at the start. If there were zero frictional forces between the skis and snow and little or no air resistance, the skier's potential energy would continually decrease in direct proportion to the increase in kinetic energy. However, frictional forces exist and they influence the magnitude of one's kinetic energy. Nevertheless, the underlining force that allows the skier to develop significant kinetic energy is the constant pull by gravity. It is this force that generates a skier's downhill velocity.

To maximize the use of the pull of gravity, a skier applies special waxing substances developed for certain weather conditions to lessen the influence of frictional forces. The skier also attempts to present a smaller frontal surface area by wearing clothing that is not only warm but tight-fitting to lessen the air resistance.

The reason is that as the skier increases speed (velocity), there is a corresponding increase in air resistance, which slows a person's acceleration down the hill.

ACTIVITIES:

1. Research the effect of gravity and resistive forces on the following activities and discuss their similarities and dissimilarities.

   a. skydiving

   b. trampolining

   c. platform diving (10 meters)

2. Describe the two most popularly used ski turns in downhill skiing and explain their effects on the skier's velocity.

FOOTBALL

CONCEPT 109: One Foot Must be in Contact with the Ground When a Player Kicks a Football

INFORMATION:

1. Newton's third law reveals that every action produces an equal and opposite reaction.

2. The emphasis in this concept is on the words "opposite reaction."

3. If one foot is in contact with the ground when forward impetus is given to an object (action), the body cannot be driven backward (reaction).

RATIONALE:

When the body is airborne at the instant a body part or an implement strikes an object, an ineffective action results because the body is subject to Newton's third law. If a foot swings forward to kick a ball while the body is in midair, the reaction at impact will drive the body backward. The reactive force from the ground that is necessary to propel the ball forward is absent and the ball travels only a short distance.

However, when the body of a kicker is in contact to the ground via the nonkicking leg, two events occur which add considerable distance to the kicked ball.

a. The mass of the body-earth combination is too great to be driven backward (reaction) as the ball is kicked forward (action).

b. The earth provides a reaction as the nonkicking leg pushes against the surface, and this reaction aids in propelling the ball.

ACTIVITIES:

Kicker A punts a football with the right foot, and the left foot is in contact with the earth. Kicker B punts a football with the right foot while the left foot is off the ground.

    a.   Which kicker will produce the longest punt?

    b.   What will happen to the body of kicker B as the kicked ball starts forward?

    c.   Why will the body of kicker A not be affected in the same manner?

    d.   What are the two forces which account for the additional length of kicker A's punt?

    e.   Which of these forces is not available to kicker B?

    f.   Why is this second force not available to kicker B?

GOLF

CONCEPT 110: The Full Golf Swing Uses an Increased Lever System to Gain Maximum Linear Velocity of the Clubhead

INFORMATION:

1. If a lever system is increased in length and the angular velocity at the axis of rotation remains the same or is also increased, there will be a corresponding increase in the linear velocity at the distal end of the lever.
2. To impart maximum acceleration to a golf ball, the clubhead must strike the ball directly through its center of gravity while traveling at peak velocity.

RATIONALE:

If a golfer has a full swing that is essentially the same for all clubs, the only basic difference in the golf swing is the length of the club (lever) and the relative angle of inclination of the clubface. Assuming that environmental conditions are ideal, the ball will travel the maximum distance when the following techniques are applied:

1. Golfer assumes a stable stance.
2. Left arm is straight, left shoulder higher than the right shoulder.
3. Clubhead is drawn back in a flattened arc and to the inside of the intended line of flight.
4. Torquing of the trunk and shoulders places these powerful muscles on stretch.
5. Left wrist is straight and firm, right wrist hyperextended, right elbow in close to the body while at the top of the swing.
6. Head is slightly turned, chin elevated to allow left shoulder to turn beneath it.
7. Downswing starts with forward (lateral) movement of the hips.
8. Shoulders, arms, and hands follow downward while hips move laterally forward.

9. Wrists begin uncocking as a result of the centrifugal force applied to the clubhead and are rolled (turned) before impact.
10. At impact, the grip is firm, the clubface at right angles to the intended direction, and the center of gravity of the clubhead directly behind the center of gravity of the ball.
11. The clubhead should be moving at its maximum velocity.

Many other factors have been omitted for the sake of brevity, but the basic elements of the swing are included. Assuming these techniques are used properly, all the golfer needs to do is ascertain his or her distance from the hole and use the proper club.

It is generally agreed that the following distances in yards can be obtained by selecting the proper club.

Driver   210-240 yards
3-wood 190-220 yards
3-iron   170-200 yards
5-iron   150-180 yards
7-iron   130-160 yards
9-iron   110-120 yards

Therefore, if the golfer can maintain the same angular velocity for all clubs, and increases the length of the lever system by swinging with a longer club, the arc becomes greater. Thus the clubhead moves through a greater distance along the arc in the same period of time. For example, if a longer club moves a distance of 2 feet in one second and a shorter club moves 1 foot in one second, the former is moving twice as fast as the latter.

ACTIVITIES:

1. Experiment hitting a golf ball with two different clubs. Take a driver and a 5-iron and hit 20 to 30 balls with each club. Take a full swing, but for every five hits, shorten your grip by "choking" down on the club. Observe any differences in the distances that the balls travel.

Name _____

Section _____

GYMNASTICS

CONCEPT 111: *Centrifugal Force (Inertia) and Centripetal Force Must Counterbalance One Another During the Performance of a Giant Swing on the Horizontal Bar*

INFORMATION:

1. **Centrifugal force** (inertia) attempts to pull an object out of its orbit. It is a force exerted away from the axis of rotation.
2. **Centripetal force** attempts to maintain an object in an orbital path. It is a force exerted toward an axis of rotation.
3. **Angular momentum** is the product of the moment of inertia and angular velocity.

RATIONALE:

When performing a giant swing on the horizontal bar, a performer must consider a number of factors, the most important being the use of the law of angular momentum.

Prior to mounting the horizontal bar, the gymnast chalks the hands to decrease the friction between the bar and the hands. Once movement is achieved, Newton's first law of motion is the governing force. Simply, it states that every object in a state of motion will continue in that state unless some external force is imposed upon the object to alter its motion. The external force in this situation is the pull of gravity.

To counteract the force of gravity and continue swinging, the gymnast must change the length of the body. Assuming a counterclockwise swing with the gymnast facing the ceiling on the upward swing and the floor on the downward swing, to increase the angular velocity on the upswing (opposing gravity), the gymnast must slightly flex at the shoulders, hips, and knees, thereby decreasing the overall length of the body. This brings the total mass parts of the body closer to the axis of rotation, thereby decreasing the gymnast's moment of inertia. If there is an

283

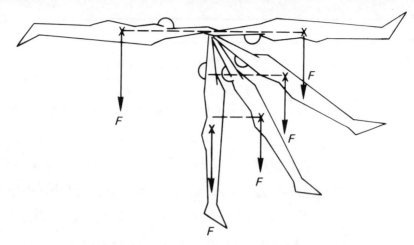

Effect of gravity on a horizontal swing.

increase in angular velocity and a corresponding decrease in moment of inertia, then the angular momentum remains relatively unchanged and the gymnast continues in the upswing without a significant loss in the speed of movement.

The opposite action occurs in the downswing. Speed is increased by the influence of gravitational pull. To decrease the effect of this force, the gymnast lengthens all body parts, thereby increasing the moment of inertia and decreasing the angular velocity while maintaining a constant angular momentum.

As the gymnast completes the swing, the inertial (centrifugal) forces are attempting to pull the gymnast away from the bar. This is why it is important for a gymnast to possess high degrees of muscular strength in the hands, wrists, arms, and shoulders to counterbalance this outward pull. Without this strength, an individual would fly off at a tangent to the swinging arc.

ACTIVITIES:

1. Analyze the giant swing in the film series produced by the Athletic Institute or some other comparable film production and note the body changes that occur during the swing. Or observe a competent performer on a gymnastic team executing a giant swing. Cite the mechanical principles involved.

2. Place yourself at the end of a human chain that is rotating while on ice skates, roller skates, or while running, and observe the effect of centripetal and centrifugal forces. Cite the mechanical principles involved.

GYMNASTICS

CONCEPT 112: A Floor Routine During the Free-Exercise Event Uses a Number of Biomechanical Concepts

INFORMATION:

1. A floor routine is an event that calls for fast and slow movements, explosive stunts and tumbling maneuvers, balancing skills, and rhythm.
2. The gymnast runs fast to gather linear momentum, goes into the air to perform specific stunts, and must land with dynamic balance.
3. To accomplish these feats, a number of biomechanical concepts are involved. They include stability, transfer of momentum, angular momentum, force production and dissipation, kinetic and potential energy, torque, and each of Newton's laws of motion.

RATIONALE:

Let us assume that during the first tumbling pass the gymnast wishes to perform a single front somersault. In the execution of this skill a number of biomechanical principles are involved. First, sufficient linear momentum has to be achieved in the run across the mat. Prior to the trick, the gymnast lowers the center of gravity to place the powerful leg extensor muscles on stretch, and checks linear velocity (forward horizontal eccentric thrust) at the extremity, uses a "punch" technique and allows the center of gravity to ride over the planted feet, then performs a powerful extensor action against the floor. The reactive force propels the gymnast upward. Because this reactive force passes posteriorly to the center of gravity (there is a slight lean at takeoff), a forward rotation occurs. The gymnast assumes a tight tuck position; this decreases the moment of inertia and increases the angular velocity, yielding sufficient angular momentum to execute a complete somersault while airborne.

Prior to landing, the gymnast untucks, thereby increasing the moment of inertia, slowing the angular velocity, and landing on the mat with slightly flexed hips, knees, and ankles to absorb the shock (force) of landing. This allows for a more gradual reduction of the kinetic energy of the "fall," reducing the force of impact. The gymnast lands with the feet together or apart depending upon what follows for the next trick.

As you can detect, in just one gymnastic trick a number of biomechanical principles came into play.

ACTIVITIES:

1. Analyze the following gymnastic tricks and cite the various biomechanical principles which apply.

   a. Front handspring on the vault.

   b. Round-off back handspring on the floor.

   c. Front double somersault dismount on rings.

2. View or observe a basic routine on the parallel bars and attempt to cite the biomechanical concepts used.

Name _____

Section _____

ICE SKATING

CONCEPT 113: A Whirling Figure Skater Uses Changing Moments of Inertia to Control Angular Velocity

INFORMATION:

1. As a figure skater whirls on the toe of one skate, the axis of rotation becomes the point in contact with the ice (the toe), and this axis extends vertically upward through the body.
2. The moment of inertia is measured from the axis of rotation for the total body to the points of the body which protrude the greatest distance from the axis.
3. Angular momentum is the product of angular velocity and moment of inertia.

RATIONALE:

At a certain point in the routine, a figure skater balances on one toe and begins to pirouette on the toe of one skate, the opposite leg no longer contacting the surface of the ice. The speed of pirouettes (angular velocity) is slow at first, but as the skater adducts the free leg and the abducted arms, angular velocity increases, To reduce angular velocity, the free leg moves away from the body, and the arms are abducted. Thus, the angular velocity is reduced to a rate where the skater can proceed to the next part of the routine.

Once the whirling action started, the skater produced no force that would explain the increase in angular velocity and the decrease that followed. The explanation lies in the change in the length of moments of inertia from the axis of rotation, the toe of the skate.

ACTIVITIES:

1. As the skater brought the free leg toward the midline and adducted the arms, what change occurred in the moment of inertia for the total body? Explain.

287

2. How did this affect the angular velocity around the toe of the skate contacting the ice? Explain.

3. As the skater abducted the arms and moved the free leg away from the midline as in an arabesque position, why did the angular velocity decrease? Explain.

STARTING

CONCEPT 114: There Are Some Motor Activities in Which the Performer Wishes to Lose Stability in Certain Starting Events

INFORMATION

1. In order to lose stability, the center of gravity must fall beyond a margin of the base of support.

2. Stability is lost rapidly when a margin of the base of support is removed.

3. Starting positions in motor skills provide for rapid loss of stability.

RATIONALE:

In motor activities such as track and swimming, a performer who has attained a position emphasizing stability after the "take your marks!" command wishes to lose that stability at the pistol shot.

During the track start, the athlete raises the hands at the pistol shot, removing the front margin of the base of support. The center of gravity is now in front of the new base of support beneath the feet. The performer immediately becomes unstable in order to begin the race.

While in the preliminary position for the racing start in swimming, the performer has the center of gravity at the extreme front margin of the base of support. Any movement of the legs, trunk, or arms will project the center of gravity beyond the front margin of the base of support. The performer then rapidly loses stability because the center of gravity becomes influenced by the pull of gravity.

ACTIVITIES:

1. The following diagram represents the base of support previous to the pistol shot for a track sprinter.

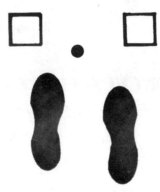

    a.   Where is the center of gravity in relation to the base of support?

    b.   How is this relationship altered when the pistol fires?

2. The following diagram represents the base of support for a general starting position for motor activities.

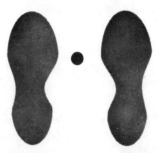

    a.   Why is the center of gravity in the middle of the base of support if this factor limits mobility?

    b.   What is the rationale for encouraging performers to have their weight on the balls of the feet in such a starting position?

SWIMMING

CONCEPT 115: Effort That Does Not Contribute to the Desired Result Acts as a Resistance

INFORMATION:

1. In the early stages of learning motor skills, performers are prone to make unnecessary movements which do not contribute to the desired result.
2. Such extra movements add to the workload, cause the performer to consume additional oxygen, and act as physiological resistance.

RATIONALE:

During imperfect performances of motor skills, inexperienced performers are apt to make unnecessary movements. Observe the thrashing of a beginning swimmer who attempts to stay afloat by performing the crawl stroke.

The problem of unnecessary movements in performing motor skills is not limited to the novice. Many swimmers employ movements that do little to produce locomotion. Examples include too high a leg kick. Lifting the arms too high and turning the body over on its side to breathe create unnecessary movements. These unnecessary movements require additional energy expenditure and place increased demands on the oxygen delivery mechanism.

ACTIVITIES:

1. A swimmer was observed while practicing the crawl stroke kick. The lower leg rose above the surface on the upstroke, and the entire leg was submerged on the downstroke. Despite an exhaustive effort, the swimmer made little forward progress. Why?

2. Why is an overly vigorous arm action inefficient for the long distance runner?

3. Swimmer A used a few slow, powerful strokes when swimming underwater. Swimmer B employed a number of very rapid strokes but could not swim as far underwater as swimmer A. Explain.

SWIMMING

CONCEPT 116: Movement Through the Water is Best Achieved by the Effective Use of a Swimmer's Arms and Legs

INFORMATION:

1. Propulsion through the water is best demonstrated by Newton's third law of motion.
2. The most effective application of force should occur when the arm is perpendicular to and directly under the body.
3. The resistance that an object creates in the water increases with the square of the velocity.

RATIONALE:

Resistance or drag must be minimized for efficient swimming. Decreasing drag can be accomplished by streamlining the body, thus reducing the total resistive surface area facing the intended direction of motion. Allowing the legs to drop too deeply in the water while kicking increases the resistive forces. If the arm recovery is too far from the trunk it not only slows the recovery rate but also causes the lower body to waggle through the water. It is important to have a high elbow recovery for improved efficiency. See the arm diagrams below.

During the recovery phase of the arm cycle when the arm is out of the water, the elbow should be elevated and flexed so that the moment of inertia of the limb is

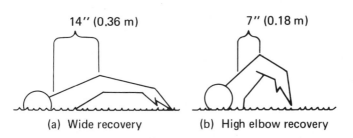

14″ (0.36 m)   7″ (0.18 m)

(a) Wide recovery   (b) High elbow recovery

decreased, thus increasing its angular velocity. This assists the speed of the arm cycle so that forward momentum is maintained. It is also important that an even speed of movement be maintained.

Proper placement of the hand and arm into the water is important. If the hand and arm initiate downward force too early after entry, there is an upward reactive force causing inefficient movement. The hand should be flexed at the wrist and the arm flexed at the elbow so that the backward push (active force) by the arm is directed backward. The hand also is positioned directly under the center of the trunk so that the backward push produces a forward push (reactive force).

As the speed of movement increases, the cost of performing the movement also increases disproportionally; in fact, the resistance created by the object increases with the square of the linear velocity. Thus, it is important to determine the appropriate terminal velocity that is specific to each swimmer. In sum, if the velocity of the forward moment is too fast, the resistive forces may result in a net negative force causing early fatigue, especially in long distance swimming events.

ACTIVITIES:

1. Using a kick board, kick vigorously with high heel recovery for one lap and then kick with proper kicking and note the difference. Explain what occurs.

2. Execute a wide arm recovery and sidearm pull for one lap then a high elbow recovery with a beneath the trunk pull and note the difference. Explain what occurs.

SWIMMING

CONCEPT 117: A Diver Can Perform More Somersaults in the Tuck Position, Fewer in the Pike Position, and Fewest in the Layout Position

INFORMATION:

1. The *moment of inertia* is measured from the distal ends of the body to the axis of motion. (Note: $I = \Sigma mr^2$.)
2. A moment of inertia is analogous to a lever. When the moment of inertia is lengthened, angular velocity decreases. The reverse is true when a moment of inertia is decreased.
3. The center of gravity of the body is the axis of motion for the total body during airborne somersaults.

RATIONALE:

A diver performing front somersaults rotates forward in the sagittal plane around an axis of motion which passes through the center of gravity. The moment of inertia for this motor skill is measured from the center of gravity to the distal point of the body. The length of the moment of inertia is inversely proportional to its angular velocity (force remaining constant). The moment of inertia for somersaults is longest in the layout position, intermediate in the pike position, and shortest in the tuck position. The angular velocity is greatest in the tuck and least in the layout, with the pike occupying the intermediate ranking. Therefore, a diver can perform more revolutions per unit of time in the tuck, fewer in the pike position, and fewest in the layout position. In sum, one changes the distribution of mass about an axis of rotation.

As the moments of inertia decrease assuming the same angular momentum, there will be a corresponding increase in angular velocities. Hence, the opportunity for increased revolutions.

ACTIVITIES:

Complete the following table.

A diver is in the air for 3 seconds. How many somersaults are possible? (360 degrees = one revolution.) (Can be answered using the ratio technique.)

POSITION	LENGTH OF MOMENT OF INERTIA	ANGULAR VELOCITY	SOMERSAULTS POSSIBLE
Layout	3 ft	120°/sec	_____
Pike	2 ft	_____	_____
Tuck	1.5 ft	_____	_____

TENNIS

CONCEPT 118: Increasing the Length of a Movement of Force Produces Stronger Joint Movements When Striking (Giving Impetus to) a Tennis Ball

INFORMATION:

1. *Moment of force* is defined as the product of the amount of force times the perpendicular distance from the axis of motion (joint) to the distal end of the moving body segment. (Note: $F \times TFA$.)

2. The distal end of a longer lever possesses greater velocity than the distal end of a shorter lever when the force moving the levers is constant. Therefore, the greater the moment of force, the greater the linear velocity at the distal end.

RATIONALE:

A ball can be struck more forcefully with a racquet held in the hand than if the palm of the hand were the striking surface. When an implement such as a tennis racket is held in the hand, its length is added to the length of the arm. This results in an increase in the moment of force for each joint which helps to move the tennis racket. The final result is an increase in linear velocity, since it is the racquet face, and not the hand, which strikes the ball.

Basically the situation is similar to increasing the length of golf clubs. If the angular velocity remains constant, and the lever is increased, the distal end of the longer lever will possess greater linear velocity.

ACTIVITIES:

1. The following stick drawing represents the arm traveling through a range of horizontal extension. Points A, B, and C represent the elbow, wrist, and finger tips.

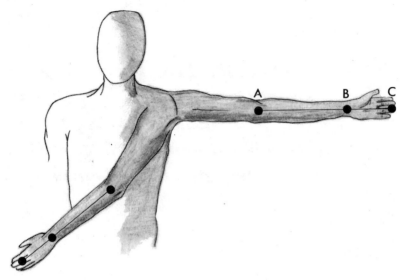

   a. Which point possesses the greatest velocity?

   b. Why?

2. Two tennis rackets are swung with equal force. Calculate the velocity of the tip of each racket. (Note: $v = d/t$.)

A	B
Length of racket = 22″	Length of racket = 26″
Length of arm + racket = 52″	Length of arm + racket = 56″
Distance racket tip travels = 9.5 feet	Distance racket tip travels = 13.5 feet
Time = .8 seconds	Time = 1.1 seconds
Velocity of racket tip = _____	Velocity of racket tip = _____

TENNIS

CONCEPT 119: Follow-Through Places the Body in a "Ready Position" to Begin the Next Tennis Skill

INFORMATION:

1. A tennis player who serves the ball and then enters the court in a "ready position" is prepared to field a serve returned by the opponent.
2. Stability may be lacking at the end of one movement and must be regained in order to perform the next movement in a sequence.
3. Follow-through at the end of one movement permits the re-establishment of stability and places the body in a position to begin the next movement in the sequence.

RATIONALE:

A tennis server must ensure proper contact with the ball and then must move rapidly onto the court to contest the point when the serve is returned. In order to accomplish the sequence of movements, the server must re-establish stability after the serve is completed and is then in a ready position to move onto the court.

The server who is off balance at the completion of the serve, will experience difficulty in moving onto the court.

Follow-through at the end of the serve provides time to control body momentum, re-establish stability, and use momentum gathered during the serve to move the body onto the court.

ACTIVITIES:

1. Explain the sequence of events after a tennis player hits a forehand shot from the right baseline corner.

2. Explain the sequence of events after a tennis player hits a backhand volley shot while at the net.

TRACK AND FIELD

CONCEPT 120: When the Body is in Free Flight, No Amount of Maneuvering of Body Parts Can Alter the Path of the Center of Gravity

INFORMATION:

1. The body becomes a projectile during jumping, leaping, bouncing, and diving activities.
2. According to Newton's first law, a force is necessary to change the path of a body in motion.
3. A body which is airborne is free from surfaces against which it could exert a force.
4. The path of the human body in flight is predetermined at the instant of takeoff.
5. A body in flight is subject to Newton's third law of action-reaction.

RATIONALE:

The path of the center of gravity of the human body in flight is predetermined at the moment of takeoff by two factors: (1) the force exerted or the velocity obtained, and (2) the angle of takeoff. Once the body is airborne, it lacks a surface against which force can be applied. No amount of maneuvering of body parts can change the predetermined path of the center of gravity.

The body in flight is subject to Newton's law of action-reaction. Any movement made on one side of the center of gravity will cause body parts on the other side of the center of gravity to move in the opposite direction.

The running long jumper makes many movements in midair. These movements have no effect upon the path of the center of gravity.

ACTIVITIES:

The following series of figures represents movements performed by a long jumper while in midair. The arrows represent the movements initiated by the jumper (action). Indicate by arrows the opposite direction movements produced by reaction.

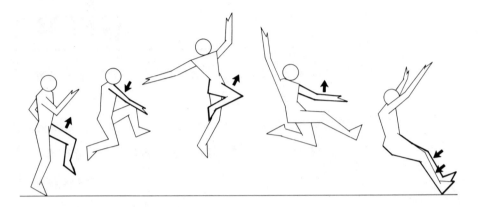

TRACK AND FIELD

CONCEPT 121: Centrifugal Force (Inertia) and Centripetal Force Must Counterbalance One Another During the Hammer Throw

INFORMATION:

1. *Centrifugal force* (inertia) attempts to pull an object out of its orbit. It is a force exerted away from an axis of rotation.

2. *Centripetal force* attempts to maintain an object in an orbital path. It is a force exerted toward an axis of rotation.

RATIONALE:

During the hammer throw, centrifugal force (inertia) exerts a pull away from the axis of rotation (the athlete). The hammer attempts to escape from its orbit around the athlete. The source of centrifugal force is the mass of the hammer.

If centrifugal force is not counterbalanced by some equal and opposite force, the hammer escapes from its orbit and becomes subject to Newton's first law. In the hammer throw, the counterbalancing force is centripetal force, provided by the tensile strength of the cable of the hammer and by the muscular strength of the athlete.

Should the athlete flex the elbows, the amount of centripetal force would increase. Centripetal force would surpass centrifugal force, and the hammer would be drawn closer to the axis of rotation. Should centrifugal force exceed centripetal force, the athlete would be forced to release the hammer. See the diagram on the next page.

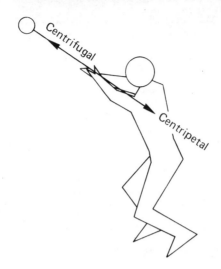

ACTIVITIES:

1. Diagram the resultant path of the hammer when it is released by the thrower or when centrifugal force overcomes centripetal force.

2. Complete the following table by supplying the source of centrifugal and centripetal forces for each activity.

ACTIVITY	SOURCE OF CENTRIPETAL FORCE	SOURCE OF CENTRIFUGAL FORCE
Hammer throw	Muscle contraction	Mass of hammer
Giant swing		
Water skiing		
Windmill softball pitch		

TRACK AND FIELD

CONCEPT 122: Hurdlers Must Minimize Their Time in the Air

INFORMATION:

1. The leg speed of the leading foot at takeoff is an important technique for clearing the hurdle properly.
2. The high point of the hurdler's center of gravity must come before the hurdle and be only slightly higher than a normal running stride.
3. A proper forward trunk lean with correct arm and leg position while clearing the hurdle ensures a rapid return to the ground.

RATIONALE:

To be successful at high hurdling it is imperative that the performer minimize clearance time over the hurdle in order to get back to the ground and maintain maximum velocity. World-class performers practice many hours perfecting their glide over the hurdles to reduce airborne time. Thus it is important for the hurdler to pass over the 3 feet, 6 inch or 1.067 meter height as rapidly as possible.

To ensure proper leading leg speed in the takeoff phase, it is necessary to initially flex the leg at the knee and hip, thereby decreasing the leg's moment of inertia and increasing the angular velocity of the lower limb. Once this is accomplished, the leg is extended at the knee and the foot is held slightly higher than the hurdle. See diagrams below.

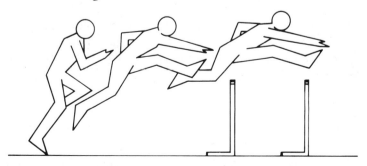

While the leading leg is thrust forward at takeoff, the upper body (trunk) flexes forward at the hurdler's center of gravity to facilitate horizontal speed. To prevent trunk rotation, the leading leg is counteracted by the opposite side arm to control Newton's third law of motion as it manifests. See diagram below.

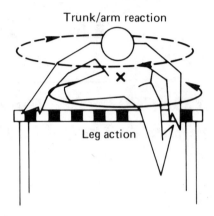

The trailing leg is abducted to the side, and flexed at the hip and knee as it passes over the hurdle, thus decreasing the moment of inertia of the trailing leg and increasing its angular velocity. See diagrams below.

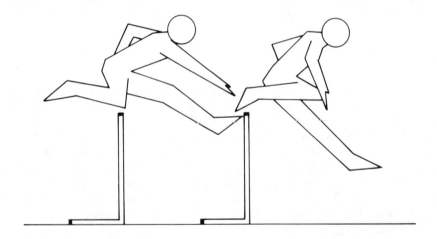

As the lead leg is forcefully driven downward once over the hurdle, the trunk is driven backwards in counteraction to the leg drive. Again, the arms counterbalance each other to prevent excessive horizontal trunk and hip rotation. See diagram on the next page.

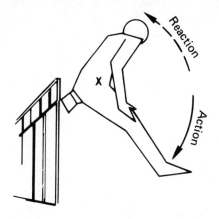

Finally the leading leg is planted on the ground and the trail leg is thrust forward to bring the first full running stride. See diagram below.

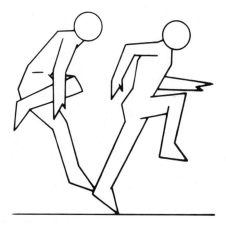

ACTIVTIES:

1. Time a group of hurdlers from takeoff to landing while they are running over the fourth hurdle, they should be at or near maximum velocity at this point.

2. Execute at least six hurdle attempts. In each situation vary the arm position, trunk lean, trailing leg position, and some other techniques. Cite the effects of the proper and improper techniques.

TRACK AND FIELD

CONCEPT 123: *The Purpose of High Jumping is to Propel the Center of Gravity to a Height Sufficient for Good Performance*

INFORMATION:

1. A person's height, muscular explosiveness, or power and position over the bar are successful ingredients in high jumping.
2. Gathering one's internal muscular forces at takeoff may be the single most important factor in jumping, because achieving maximal vertical lift velocity is essential for good performance.

RATIONALE:

An efficient and effective high jump must possess the following: a proper approach, appropriate speed during approach, vertical lift during takeoff, and correct position over the bar. The discussion that follows emphasizes these points while explaining the conventional straddle jump and the newly developed flop technique.

The direction of one's approach is a matter of personal preference. However, research indicates that an approach too parallel to the bar will cause the jumper to travel along the bar. An approach directly at the bar may cause the athlete to jump prematurely and thus fail to allow adequate time for the free leg swing. According to experts in sport biomechanics, the recommended angle of approach for most high jump techniques is between 20 and 30 degrees. This apparently allows for proper free leg swing (transferring angular momentum) and for generation of force at takeoff (impulse).

The speed of the approach is related to a number of factors—the height of the bar, the time necessary for proper positioning at takeoff, and the strength of the individual. It has been noted that world-class jumpers run at speeds of from 15 to 16 mph.

Setting up for the takeoff while employing sound biomechanical principles to achieve maximum vertical lift velocity is the single most important factor in high jumping. During the final steps of the straddle jump, the individual lowers the center, leans backwards, and plants the lead leg at about a 45-degree angle with the ground, thereby checking linear velocity and starting vertical eccentric thrust. The impulse, the product of time and muscular force, becomes significant. In high jumping it is important to generate greater muscular force than to stay on the ground for extended periods. In fact, researchers claim that the higher the jump, the less time one stays on the ground. See diagrams below.

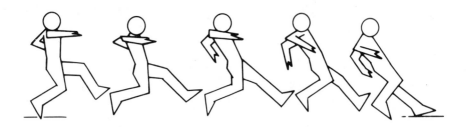

Next, the free leg swings forward. To increase the speed of the limb, the knee is flexed to decrease the moment of inertia and increase its angular velocity. The planted leg flexes slightly at the knee and hip not only to absorb the force from the speed of the approach but also to place the powerful extensor muscles on stretch. As the free leg now fully extended transfers its momentum to the rest of the body, both arms swing forward and upward to impact vertical acceleration and add transfer of momentum to influence vertical velocity. See diagrams below.

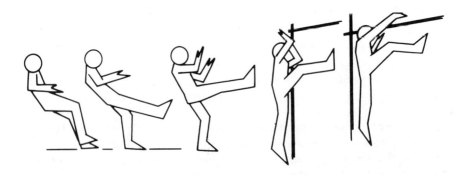

It should be pointed out that while the individual is airborne and going over the bar the flight path is predetermined; nothing can alter it in the air. Any action will cause an equal and opposite reaction. However, one can change body position around the center of gravity and change the moment of inertia at the body, thus either increasing or decreasing angular velocity of body parts while airborne. Rotating about the longitudinal axis with the stomach facing the bar enables the trailing leg and arm to clear the bar. See diagrams on the next page.

310

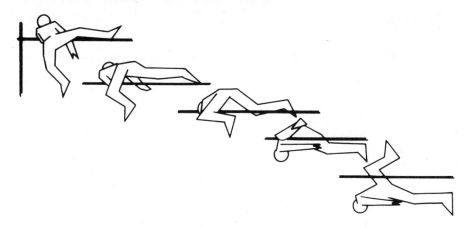

In the flop technique the approach is more abrupt. The same checking of linear velocity for developing vertical eccentric thrust, takes place but the magnitude is not nearly as great as in the straddle technique.

Because there is a sharp turn during the last few strides on the approach to the bar and because it is the inside left leg that is used to rotate the jumper clockwise, the execution depends on the centrifugal force that is generated by this pathway. The jumper then is propelled off at a tangent to the arc. It is this activity that is used to develop the jumper's vertical lift.

The clockwise rotation of the inside leg imparts a transfer of angular momentum to the body and twists the body so the jumper's back faces the bar. While the jumper is airborne over the bar there is a downward action by the trunk causing a downward counter reaction by the legs. This action creates a hyperextended position and also diminishes any further twisting along the longitudinal axis; it also lowers the center of gravity. In fact, this is one of the significant differences between the flop and straddle techniques. The body does not have to go as high in the flop technique. To land safely the jumper lifts the legs (action) once they clear the bar to cause the trunk (reaction) to remain parallel for proper landing. See diagrams below.

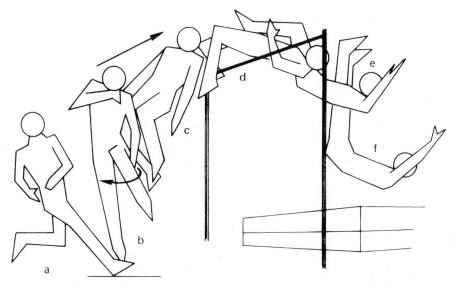

ACTIVITIES:

1. Compare the following high jump techniques biomechanically: flop versus scissors.

2. Compare the following high jump techniques biomechanically: straddle versus western roll.

VOLLEYBALL

CONCEPT 124: The Forearm Bump Pass is an Example of Receiving Impetus (Momentum of an Object)

INFORMATION:

1. A large, flat surface is created to assist in dissipating the kinetic energy of an oncoming ball.
2. The forearms collapse slightly and the person lowers the center of gravity by flexing at the knees to reduce the ball's kinetic energy.
3. The individual attempts to position him- or herself so as to increase the base of support in line with the direction of the oncoming ball.

RATIONALE:

The forearm bump pass is an important volleyball technique because it is the primary technique used when receiving the ball hit by the opponent.

Because the ball usually travels at high speeds, it is necessary to use a number of techniques to try to gradually reduce the kinetic energy of the oncoming ball. Increasing the exposed surface area (both forearms) assists the individual in dissipating the kinetic energy of the ball. At the moment of contact, the forearms collapse slightly to reduce the kinetic energy by absorbing the oncoming force. See diagram below.

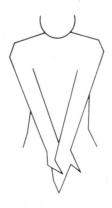

313

To increase stability while receiving the ball and ensure an effective pass after contact, the player attempts to position him- or herself in front of the line of direction of the ball. The player lowers the center of gravity by flexing at the knees to assist in absorbing some of the force of the ball. The feet also are spread in the direction to increase the base of support and to execute a proper bump pass to a teammate. See diagrams below.

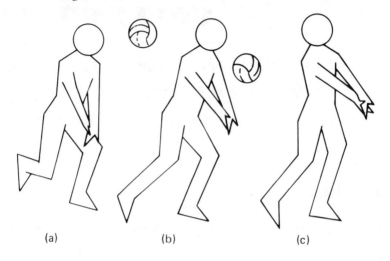

(a) (b) (c)

ACTIVITIES:

1. Compare the offensive bump pass with the defensive dig pass.

2. Cite any other biomechanical concepts that are important for execution of the bump pass.

Name _____

Section _____

VOLLEYBALL

CONCEPT 125: Spiking the Ball is an Example of Giving Impetus to an Object

INFORMATION:

1. Applying force directly through the center of gravity of a ball will cause the ball to move in a straight path; applying force outside the center of gravity creates an eccentric thrust and causes the ball to spin.

2. Hitting the ball with an increased surface area aids in the application of force.

3. Developing muscular effort (force) and applying it over a longer period of time increases the acceleration of the ball (impulse).

RATIONALE:

The objective of the spike technique in volleyball is to generate maximum acceleration and proper placement in the opponent's court. Many factors come into play in executing this skill. It is necessary to obtain maximum height on the jump, to generate sufficient velocity in the striking hand, and to effectively contact the ball for proper placement.

The height of the vertical jump is an important aspect of the skill. In preparation, the player lowers the center of gravity, places the powerful extensor muscles on stretch, and positions both arms behind the back. During upward thrust, the arms are forcefully accelerated upward for not only a proper transfer of momentum, but also to increase the force applied against the floor to bring about greater reaction force for the vertical lift.

As the spiker approaches maximum vertical height, the trunk rotates toward the striking arm. The striking arm is placed in abduction and horizontal extension at the shoulder and flexion at the elbow. This decreases the moment of inertia of the arm, thereby increasing angular velocity at the shoulder. A powerful forward action (inward rotation of the arm and extension at the elbow) of the striking arm is employed. See diagrams below.

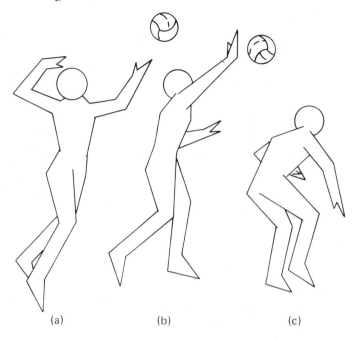

(a)   (b)   (c)

To maximize ball acceleration, three additional points should be mentioned. First, resultant linear acceleration occurs when force is directed through the center of gravity of the ball. In this situation, the applied force is directed downward into the opponent's court. Second, increasing the time of force application (without violating the carry rule) or increasing the impulse will assist the spiker in generating appropriate acceleration. Third, increasing the striking surface (open hand) increases the effectiveness of force application. However, when the spiker wishes to impart spin to make it more difficult for the opponent to return the ball, force applied outside the center of gravity will impart spin causing the ball to curve into the court through the principle of eccentric thrust.

ACTIVITIES:

1. Cite another sport form skill that is very similar to the overhead spike in volleyball. Describe and compare its biomechanical principles with that of the spike technique.

2. How is the overhead serve in volleyball different from the overhead spike and how are they alike?

WRESTLING

CONCEPT 126: The Use of Levers is Important to Successful Wrestling Techniques

INFORMATION:

1. All three types of levers are used in wrestling.
2. When muscular strength and/or explosiveness is needed, second-class levers are selected.
3. When speed and range of motion is essential, third-class levers are used.

RATIONALE:

Wrestling as a contact sport involves manipulating the actions of another person and frequently calls upon the use of the leverage system for the execution of many offensive and defensive maneuvers. As stated in previous concepts, a first-class lever can be mechanically advantageous for speed at the expense of force or vice versa depending on the placement of the fulcrum. However, a second-class lever is always mechanically beneficial to force production at the expense of speed and range of movement. A third-class lever always benefits speed and range of motion at the expense of force production.

When the offensive (top) wrestler applies a side-cradle maneuver on a prone defensive (bottom) wrestler, a first-class lever is used. The left arm is placed around the opponent's head and the right arm around the rear leg. The head is placed into the side of the opponent and the arms simultaneously pull toward one another using the head as the fulcrum, thus establishing a force-fulcrum-resistance relationship.

The use of a half-nelson in wrestling is essential and becomes a powerful maneuver because it establishes a second-class lever. When the left hand is placed under the opponent's left arm and on the opponent's head, a force-resistance-fulcrum relationship is created. The muscular force begins at the shoulder region, and the fulcrum is the hand placed on the opponent's head; between the shoulder and hand the opponent's arm resists the force. The maneuver is similar to the example of a crowbar being placed under the side of a car in an attempt to roll the car over on its side. The speed in both cases is unimportant; it is the cranking action

317

by a slow deliberate muscular effort that will turn the defensive wrestler over on the back or the car to its side.

The single-leg takedown attempt is one of the most frequently used skills in wrestling. The attacking wrestler often has the opponent's leg in the air and is trying to force the opponent to the mat for control. This maneuver is an excellent example of the use of a third-class lever. When the attacking wrestler controls the opponent's foot (fulcrum point), applies force above the ankle but below the knee (force point), and attempts to rotate the wrestler (resistance) to the mat, a fulcrum-force-resistance relationship is established and a third-class lever created. The force does not need to be of great magnitude but when applied properly while allowing the opponent to rotate about the airborne foot, the opponent is rapidly rotated to the mat. Thus speed is gained at the expense of force.

ACTIVITIES:

1. Select and describe three fundamental wrestling skills that would use each of the three classes of levers.
    a. First-class lever skill

    b. Second-class lever skill

    c. Third-class lever skill

GLOSSARY

Acceleration: The rate of change of velocity.

Action potential: A marked change in the electrical state of the cell.

Adaptation of stress: A phenomenon whereby one misaligned body segment forces adjacent segments out of alignment.

Aerobic exercises: Exercises that require the consumption of oxygen.

Aerodynamic drag force: A fluid force that opposes the motion of an object through air.

Aerodynamic lift force: A fluid force acting perpendicular to the flow direction of an object possessing a lift-producing configuration.

Agonist: A prime mover; a muscle that produces most of the force needed to move a bone.

Anaerobic metabolism: The production of cellular energy in which chemicals other than oxygen are consumed.

Anatomical position: One in which an individual assumes the position of military attention with the palms of the hands facing forward.

Angle of pull of muscle: The angle formed between the line of pull of a contracting muscle and the plane of the bone that is moved.

Angle of takeoff: The angle formed between the line of flight of an object and the surface from which that object departs.

Angular momentum: An object's rotational inertia times its angular velocity.

Angular motion: The movement occurring when an object rotates around an axis that is within the mass of the object.

Angular velocity: The rate at which an object travels in an angular path.

Antagonist: A muscle whose action opposes the motion occurring at a joint.

Assistant mover: A muscle that aids a prime mover in overcoming a great resistance.

Axis of motion: A fulcrum; a fixed point or line about which angular motion occurs.

Base of support: The points in contact with the supporting surfaces and the two-dimensional area between those points of contact.

Biomechanics: The study of mechanics and its application to human movement.

Bipennate: The converging of fascicles to both sides of a central tendon like the plumes of a feather.

Cardinal plane: Any plane that divides the body into two equally sized portions.

Center of gravity: A point about which all parts of the body will balance. A hypothetical point in the body where all of the weight of the body is centered.

Centrifugal force: A special application of the law of inertia; the force that seemingly attempts to pull an object out of its orbit.

Centripetal force: The force that attempts to maintain an object in an orbital path.

Coefficient of friction: A ratio of the force needed to start or stop an object in motion and the force holding the object against the surface.

Concentric contraction: The contraction of a muscle as it shortens from its resting length.

Curvilinear motion: Movement occurring when an object follows a curved path or an orbit around an external axis.

Cutaneous receptor: Sensory bodies in the skin that are stimulated by changes in the external environment.

Displacement: A change in an object's position in space.

Distal: A part that is further from the body center.

Dynamics: The mechanical study of objects in motion.

Dynamic stability: The state of possessing equilibrium while in motion.

Eccentric contraction: The gradual lengthening against resistance of a concentrically contracted muscle.

Eccentric thrust: A force passing through an object at some point other than its center of gravity.

Efficiency: The ratio of work output over work input.

Exteroceptive reflex: An automatic act triggered by stimuli from the external environment.

Fascicle: A collection of individual muscle fibers (cells) bounded by a tight, dense covering of connective tissue.

Fast-twitch fiber: Skeletal muscle fibers containing large quantities of glycolytic enzymes essential for the production of rapid contractions.

Feedback: Knowledge of results of a performance.

First-class lever: A simple machine that has its fulcrum at some intermediate location between its resistance point and its force point.

Foot-pound: The amount of work accomplished when one pound of resistance is moved a distance of one foot.

Force: A push or pull exerted against a resistance.

Force arm: In a lever system, the linear distance from the force point to the axis of motion (fulcrum).

Force point: The point on a lever where a force is exerted in an attempt to move the lever.

Friction: The resistance to motion created by a contact between two surfaces.

Frontal plane: An imaginary surface passing through the body from side to side dividing the body into anterior and posterior portions.

Fulcrum: The axis of motion (rotation) in a lever system.

Fusiform muscle: The parallel arrangement of fascicles with the longitudinal axis of the muscle, finishing at both ends in tendons.

Glycolytic sequence: A complex series of chemical reactions that systematically dissolve sugar molecules.

Helping synergists: Muscles that cancel out one another's undesired movement, thus allowing one another's desired movement to occur.

Horizontal plane: An imaginary surface passing through the body, parallel to the floor, and dividing the body into superior and inferior portions.

Hydrodynamic force: A fluid force that opposes the motion of an object through the water and consists of surface (skin friction), profile drag (form drag), and wave drag.

Impetus: A force applied to an object (resistance) or person that results in giving momentum to an object or in receiving the momentum of an object or person.

Impulse: The product of force times time of application.

Inertia: The tendency of an object to remain at rest or in uniform motion in a straight line.

Isokinetic contraction: A contraction in which a muscle shortens or lengthens but maintains a constant speed throughout the movement.

Isometric contraction: A contraction in which a muscle retains its length, but increases its tension.

Isotonic contraction: A contraction in which a muscle fiber shortens.

Kinematics: The description of moving objects without regard to the forces causing their motion; a division of dynamics.

Kinesthesis: The perception of muscle movement and the relative alignment of the performer's body parts in space.

Kinetic energy: The ability of an object to perform work because it is in motion.

Kinetics: The description of moving objects with regard to the forces causing their motion; a division of dynamics.

Lever: A bony segment that moves around an axis of motion (fulcrum).

Linear velocity: The rate at which an object travels in a translatory (linear) path.

Line of muscle pull: A line that lies between the attachments of a muscle.

Locomotion: Movement occurring when the human body provides the force necessary to produce motion.

Mass: The result of dividing the weight of an object by a constant number (at sea level, 32) representing the force of gravity.

Mechanical advantage: A ratio of the amount of resistance overcome compared with the amount of energy expended.

Mid position: A position of the hands in which the palms face one another.

Mobility: The state of being capable of movement.

Moment of force: The product of the amount of force applied to a lever multiplied by the perpendicular distance from the force point to the distal end of the lever. ($F \times TFA$)

Moment of inertia: The product of the amount of resistance overcome, multiplied by the perpendicular distance from the distal end of the lever, to the axis of motion (fulcrum). ($I = \Sigma mr^2$)

Momentum: The product of the mass of an object multiplied by its velocity.

Motion: A change of position.

Multipennate: The converging of fascicles to many central tendons, as in the deltoideus muscle.

Muscle spindle: A proprioceptor, a sensor for the kinesthetic sense that is stimulated when skeletal muscle is stretched.

Myoglobin: Muscle hemoglobin; a protein compound capable of combining chemically with oxygen.

Nonrotatory component: The portion of a force or a resistance that does not produce movement at an axis of motion (joint).

Oxidative process: A complex series of chemical reactions in which electrons are "freed" from the foodstuffs we take into our bodies.

Pectoral girdle: An anatomical unit consisting of the clavicle, scapula, and the humerus.

Pelvic girdle: An anatomical unit consisting of the left and right innominate bones (ilium, ischium, pubis) and the sacrum.

Pennate muscle: The converging of fascicles to one side of a tendon running longitudinally throughout the muscle.

Perception: The process of receiving and interpreting external and internal stimuli.

Periphery: The external margin of an object or an area.

Perpendicular: At a right angle to.

Physiological advantage: The physiological ability of a muscle to contract. Muscles are at their greatest physiological advantage when at or stretched slightly beyond the resting length.

Plane: A level and flat surface that is often imaginary.

Points of contact: The parts of the body (or object) that are in contact with a supporting surface.

Potential energy: The ability of an object to perform work by virtue of its position.

Power: The quantity of work produced in a given period of time.

Prime mover: An agonist, a muscle which produces most of the force that moves a bone.

Pronated hands: A position in which the palms face rearward in the anatomical position.

Prone: A body position in which the face is down.

Proprioceptive reflex: Movement triggered by a special receptor sensitive to changes in body position.

Proprioceptors: Receptors that are stimulated by changes in body position or the alignment of body parts.

Proximal: A body part that is closer to the body center.

Rectilinear motion: Movement occurring when an object follows a straight line.

Resistance: An opposing force to be overcome.

Resistance arm: In a lever system, the linear distance from the resistance point to the axis of motion (fulcrum).

Resistance point: The center of gravity of the moving portion of the body lever.

Resting length: The length of a muscle when that muscle's body segment is in the anatomical position.

Rotation: Angular movement, motion around a fixed axis of motion.

Rotatory component: The portion of a force or a resistance that produces movement at an axis of motion (fulcrum).

Sagittal plane: An imaginary surface passing through the body from front to back, dividing the body into left and right portions.

Second-class lever: A simple machine that has its resistance point at some intermediate position between its fulcrum and its force point.

Shunt muscle: Has its upper attachment nearer the joint upon which it acts than is true of its lower attachment. Most of its force is nonrotatory and stabilizes the joint spanned.

Sliding friction: The resistance to motion created by contact between two surfaces which are free to slide.

Slow-twitch fibers: Skeletal muscle fibers containing large amount of myoglobin and oxidative enzymes essential for the production of sustained contractions.

Spurt muscle: Has its lower attachments nearer the joint upon which it acts than is true of its upper attachment. Most of its force is rotary and produces motion.

Stability: Possessing equilibrium, the ability to resist a force which could cause motion.

Stabilizer: A muscle that fixes one bony segment so that movement can occur in a bone articulating at that segment.

Starting friction: The resistance to motion created by the contact between two surfaces; must be overcome before one of the surfaces can move.

Static stability: The ability to resist a force that could set an object in motion.

Statics: The mechanical study of objects in their nonmoving states.

Stretch reflexes: An automatic contracting of a skeletal muscle that has become stretched; a postural reflex.

Supinated hands: A position in which the palms face forward in the anatomical position.

Supine: A position in which the body is lying in a face-up position.

Taut: The condition of being tightly drawn.

Third-class lever: A simple machine having its force point at some intermediate position between its resistance point and its fulcrum.

Torque: A twist exerted around an axis of motion.

Translatory motion: Movement in which an object follows a straight path or a circular path, sometimes around an external axis of motion.

True force arm: The perpendicular distance from the line of pull of a muscle to the axis of motion.

True resistance arm: The perpendicular distance from the line of pull of a resistance to the axis of motion.

True synergist: A muscle whose contraction cancels out the undesired movement of a primer mover (agonist).

Unipennate: *See* pennate muscle.

Velocity: The rate of change of motion.

Visual cues: Perceived visual stimuli which contribute to equilibrium and/or performance.

Weight: The effect of the earth's gravitational pull on an object's mass.

Work: The process of exerting a force which moves a resistance through a distance. Heat is a by-product of work.

DATE DUE